2010 EDITION

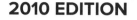

P9-CKQ-669

Nursing's Social Policy Statement

THE **Essence** OF THE **Profession**

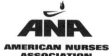

AMERICAN NURSES ASSOCIATION

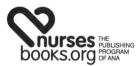

nurses books.org THE PUBLISHING PROGRAM OF ANA

American Nurses Association
Silver Spring, Maryland
2010

Library of Congress Cataloging-in-Publication data

American Nurses Association.
 Nursing's social policy statement : the essence of the profession / American Nurses
Association. — 3rd ed.
 p. ; cm.
Includes bibliographical references and index.
 ISBN-13: 978-1-55810-270-5 (softcover)
 ISBN-10: 1-55810-270-1 (softcover)
 ISBN-13: 978-1-55810-2866 (eBook, PDF format)
 ISBN-13: 978-1-55810-360-3 (eBook, EPUB format)
 ISBN-13: 978-1-55810-361-9 (eBook, Mobipocket format)
 1. Nursing. 2. Nursing—Philosophy. 3. Nursing—Practice. 4. Nursing—Social aspects. I. Title.
[DNLM: 1. Philosophy, Nursing—Guideline. 2. Nurse's Role—Guideline. 3. Nursing—standards—Guide-
line. 4. Social Responsibility—Guideline. WY 86 A512n 2010]
 RT82.A59 2010
 610.73—dc22

                       2010019423

The American Nurses Association (ANA) is a national professional association. This ANA publication—
Nursing's Social Policy Statement: The Essence of the Profession—reflects the thinking of the nursing
profession on various issues and should be reviewed in conjunction with state board of nursing policies
and practices. State law, rules, and regulations govern the practice of nursing, while *Nursing's Social
Policy Statement: The Essence of the Profession* guides nurses in the application of their professional
skills and responsibilities.

Published by Nursesbooks.org
The Publishing Program of ANA
www.Nursesbooks.org

American Nurses Association
8515 Georgia Avenue, Suite 400
Silver Spring, MD 20910-3492
1-800-274-4ANA
www.NursingWorld.org

DESIGN AND TYPESETTING: David Fox, AURAS Design, Silver Spring, MD
PRINTING: Harris LithoGraphics, Inc., Landover, MD
EDITORIAL SERVICES: Grammarians, Inc., Washington, DC: Francis Taylor (copyediting);
Kelly Saxton (proofreading); Gina Wiatrowski (indexing)

ISBN-13: 978-1-55810-270-5   SAN: 851-3481   45K   07/2011R

First printing: June 2010. Second printing: July 2011.

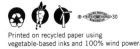

Printed on recycled paper using
vegetable-based inks and 100% wind power.

Contents

Contributors

Revision of the Social Policy Statement Workgroup, 2009–2010

Catherine E. Neuman, MSN, RN, NEA-BC – Co-Chair
John F. Dixon, MSN, RN, NE-BC – Co-Chair

Bette K. Idemoto, PhD, RN, CCRN, ACNS-BC
Pamela A. Kulbok, DNSc, RN, PHCNS-BC
Jackie R. Pfeifer, MSN, RN, APRN, CCNS
Cheryl-Ann Resha, EdD, MSN, RN
Sue Sendelbach, PhD, RN, CCNS, FAAN
Ann O'Sullivan, MSN, RN, NE-BC, CNE
Kathleen M. White, PhD, RN, CNAA-BC

ANA Staff, 2009–2010

Carol J. Bickford, PhD, RN-BC – Content editor
Katherine C. Brewer, MSN, RN – Content editor
Maureen E. Cones, Esq. – Legal counsel
Yvonne Humes, MSA – Project coordinator
Eric Wurzbacher – Project editor

Congress on Nursing Practice and Economics, 2008–2010

CHAIR
Kathleen M. White, PhD, RN, CNAA-BC

VICE-CHAIR
Ann M. O'Sullivan, MSN, RN, NE-BC, CNE

Susan A. Albrecht, PhD, RN, FAAN

Mary L. Behrens, MSN, RN, FNP-C

Carolyn Baird, MBA, MEd, RN-BC, CARN-AP, CCDP-D-Diplomate
International Nurses Society on Addictions (INSA)

Carola M. Bruflat, RNC, MSN, WHNP-BC/FNP-BC
Association of Women's Health, Obstetrics and Neonatal Nurses (AWHONN)

Garry Brydges, MSN, ACNP-BS, CRNA

Stephanie Davis Burnett, MSN, RN, ACNSpBC, CRRN
Association of Rehabilitation Nurses (ARN)

Mary Eileen Callan, MS, RN, FNP-BC

Myra C. Carmon, EdD, RN, CPNP

Robin Chard, PhD, RN, CNOR
Association of periOperative Registered Nurses (AORN)

Thomas Coe, PhD, RN, NEA-BC, FACHE

John F. Dixon, MSN, RN, NE-BC
American Association of Critical-Care Nurses (AACN)

William R. Donovan, MA, RN

Merilyn Douglass, ARNP, MSN

Bette M. Ferree, MSN, RN, FNP-BC

Susan Foster, MSN, RN, FNP-BC

Lisa A. Gorski, MS, HHCNS-BC, CRNI, FAAN
Infusion Nurses Society (INS)

Janet Y. Harris, MSN, RN, CNAA-BC

Kimberly A. Hickey, MSN, APRN-BC

Debra Hobbins, MSN, APRN

Patricia L. Holloman, RN, BSN, CNOR

Patricia K. Howard, PhD, RN, CEN
Emergency Nurses Association (ENA)

Sally Burrows-Hudson, MS, RN, CNN
American Nephrology Nurses Association (ANNA)

Bette K. Idemoto, PhD, RN, CCRN, ACNS-BC

Sandra Gracia Jones, PhD, ARNP, CS-C, ACRN, FAAN

Beverly Jorgenson, RNC, MSN, NNP

David M. Keepnews, PhD, JD, RN, FAAN

Patricia L. Keller, MSN, RN, NE-BC

Patrick E. Kenny, EdD, RN-BC, ACRN, APRN-PMH, NE-C
Association of Nurses in AIDS Care (ANAC)

Linda Riazi-Kermani, RN, BSN, CEN

Robin R. Potter-Kimball, MS, RN, CNS-BC

Jane Kirschling, DNS, RN
American Association of Colleges of Nursing (AACN)

Pamela A. Kulbok, DNSc, RN, PHCNS-BC

Kathleen G. Lawrence, MSN, RN, CWOCN
Wound Ostomy and Continence Nurses Society (WOCN)

Carla A. B. Lee, PhD, ARNP-BC, CNAA, FAAN

Lori Lioce, MSN, FNP-BC

Jennifer H. Matthews, PhD, ACNS-BC

Sara A. McCumber, RN, CNP, CNS

Peter T. Mitchell, MSN, RN, CNP, APRN-BC

Karen Leone-Natale, RN, BSN

Pamela Sue Neal, MSN-NA, RN, FNP, APRN-BC

Catherine E. Neuman, MSN, RN, NEA-BC

Linda L. Olson, PhD, RN, NEA-BC

Jackie R. Pfeifer, MSN, APRN, RN, CCNS

Theresa A. Posani, MS, RN, CNS, APRN-BC, CCRN, CNE

Elizabeth Poster, PhD, RN, FAAN

Susan E. Reinarz, MSN, RN, NNP-BC
National Association of Neonatal Nurses (NANN)

Cheryl-Ann Resha, EdD, MSN, RN
National Association of School Nurses (NASN)

Patricia Schlosser, RN, BSN

Cheryl K. Schmidt, PhD, RN, CNE, ANEF

Sue Sendelbach, PhD, RN, CCNS
National Association of Clinical Nurse Specialists (NACNS)

Nancy Shirley, PhD, RN

Joanna Sikkema, MSN, ARNP, FAHA
Preventive Cardiovascular Nurses Association (PCNA)

Elaine L. Smith, MSN, MBA, RN, CNAA
National Nursing Staff Development Organization (NNSDO)

Karen J. Stanley, MSN, RN, AOCN, FAAN
Oncology Nursing Society (ONS)

Thomas E. Stenvig, PhD, RN, MPH, CNAA

Mary Mason Wyckoff, PhD, MSN, ACNP-BC, FNP-BC, NNP, CCNS, CCRN

About the Workgroup

John F. Dixon, MSN, RN, NE-BC
Director, The Center for Nursing Education and Research, Baylor University Medical Center, Dallas TX

Mr. Dixon has over 25 years of nursing experience in critical care, education, management, administration, quality, innovation, and research in hospital practice, academic, and industry settings. Recent activities include nursing research and the development professional nursing practice models and their integration into clinical practice and operations. He has served on the American Association of Critical-Care Nurses' national board, and been the AACCN organizational liaison representative to ANA.

Bette K. Idemoto, PhD, RN, CCRN, ACNS-BC
Cardiovascular Clinical Nurse Specialist, University Hospitals Case Medical Center, Cleveland, OH

An experienced CNS, Dr. Idemoto has almost 40 years of nursing in acute and critical care, and has been educator, mentor, and presenter on a wide range of clinical topics. Her area of study includes delirium in the critically ill. She has encouraged participation among staff nurses in research scholarship, promoting nursing research through the coordination of evidence-based practice conferences, project development, and a nursing research internship program. Dr. Idemoto has served at the local, state and national levels of the ANA and other nursing organizations.

Pamela A. Kulbok, DNSc, RN, PHCNS-BC
Associate Professor of Nursing and Public Health Sciences; Coordinator of Community/Public Health Leadership, University of Virginia, School of Nursing, Charlottesville, VA

Dr. Kulbok's nursing career has included the U.S. Navy, a visiting nurse service, directing a hospital-based home health agency, and teaching undergraduate and graduate courses in public health nursing, health promotion research, and nursing knowledge development. She is the Principle Investigator of an inter-professional, cross-institution, community-based research project in substance use prevention. An active ANA member, she has held leadership roles in two public health nursing organizations.

Catherine E. Neuman, MSN, RN, NEA-BC
Nurse Consultant, Marion, IL

With over 30 years of practice as a chief nursing executive, Ms. Neuman has been director of nursing education, an infection control nurse, and a staff nurse in acute care hospitals. She has been a leader in and an active member of ANA and the Illinois Nurses Association; her state-level work includes nurse representative to the hospital licensing board. She is involved in both the ANCC Magnet Nursing Recognition Program as an appraiser and mentor, and in ANCC's Pathway to Excellence Program as a reviewer. She is presently a nurse consultant and an active parish nurse and staff nurse at a free clinic.

Jackie R. Pfeifer, MSN, RN, CCNS, APRN
Advance Practice Registered Nurse, Interventional Radiology, Marshfield Clinic, Marshfield, WI

As a clinical nurse specialist, Mrs. Pfeifer has over 10 years of experience in patient care, which has included specialty practice in medical–cardiology, surgical intensive care, and ambulatory care. She is an active member of the Wisconsin Nurses Association and American Association of Critical Care Nurses. She currently sits on the board as a Director-at-Large for the Center for American Nurses. Mrs. Pfeifer has a passion for the promoting access and the improvement in the quality of care provided at all levels of care.

Cheryl-Ann Resha, EdD, MSN, RN
Director, School Health and Nutrition Programs, Connecticut Department of Education; Adjunct Professor, University of Hartford; College of Education, Nursing and Health Professions

A nurse administrator and nurse educator working in the field of public policy and pediatric health and wellness, Dr. Resha has over 30 years experience of clinical practice, administration, and education aimed at improving the health and well-being of children and their families. Her more recent work in the state government involves advocating for school health programs, safe and healthy school environments, and such school nursing practice issues as competency and the roles of school nurses in public health and community nursing. In this role, she works with many state and national professional organizations.

Sue Sendelbach, PhD, RN, CCNS, FAHA
Director of Nursing Research and Clinical Nurse Specialist at Abbott Northwestern Hospital, Minneapolis, MN

Dr. Sendelbach is a nurse researcher and a clinical nurse specialist in critical care with 34 years of nursing experience. She has worked in the area of cognition of cardiovascular patients and delirium of hospitalized patients, and is an advocate for evidence-based practice in patient care. She is past president of the National Association of Clinical Nurse Specialists and the book editor for *Clinical Nurse Specialist: The Journal for Advanced Nursing Practice.*

Ann O'Sullivan, MSN, RN, NE-BC, CNE
Assistant Dean, Associate Professor, Blessing-Rieman College of Nursing, Quincy, IL

With over 35 years experience as a nurse educator and nurse administrator, with current certification as Nurse Educator and Nurse Executive, Ms. O'Sullivan has long been active in nursing and health care at the national and state level. Her national-level work includes Sigma Theta Tau and numerous contributions to developing and advocating for ANA's standards and guidelines. In addition to roles in such Illinois Nurses Association efforts as workforce advocacy and health policy, she has served on state-level groups on nursing resources and safety, and is now the nurse representative on its board of health.

Kathleen M. White, PhD, RN, NEA-BC, FAAN
Associate Professor, Johns Hopkins School of Nursing, Department of Health Systems and Outcomes; Director, Doctor of Nursing (DNP) Program

Dr. White has been involved at many levels with graduate nursing education the Johns Hopkins University School of Nursing. As a clinical nurse specialist at the Johns Hopkins Hospital, she is a member of the collaborative SON/JHH team that has developed nursing evidence-based practice model and guidelines. She also maintains a faculty practice appointment at Howard County General Hospital as nurse research liaison focusing on EBP initiatives. Her practice leadership roles include such Maryland state-level issues as hospital performance evaluation and patient safety, and nationally, including leadership and other roles in ANA's standards and guidelines work.

About the American Nurses Association

The American Nurses Association (ANA) is the only full-service professional organization representing the interests of the nation's 3.1 million registered nurses through its constituent/state nurses associations and its organizational affiliates. The ANA advances the nursing profession by fostering high standards of nursing practice, promoting the rights of nurses in the workplace, project-ing a positive and realistic view of nursing, and by lobbying the Congress and regulatory agencies on health care issues affecting nurses and the public.

About Nursesbooks.org,
The Publishing Program of ANA

Nursesbooks.org publishes books on ANA core issues and programs, including ethics, leadership, quality, specialty practice, advanced practice, and the pro-fession's enduring legacy. Best known for the foundational documents of the profession on nursing ethics, scope and standards of practice, and social policy, Nursesbooks.org is the publisher for the professional, career-oriented nurse, reaching and serving nurse educators, administrators, managers, and research-ers as well as staff nurses in the course of their professional development.

Nursing's Social Policy Statement: An Overview

"Nursing is the pivotal health care profession, highly valued for its specialized knowledge, skill, and caring in improving the health status of the public and ensuring safe, effective, quality care."

(ANA, 2002)

This revision of *Nursing's Social Policy Statement* is the culmination of an extensive review process that also included a long public comment period. It builds on previous editions, especially the original 1980 document. The work describes the essence of the profession by discussing nursing as a profession that is both valued within a society and uniquely accountable to that society. The definition of nursing follows and describes contemporary nursing practice. A more detailed discussion of practice is presented in the sections about the scope and standards of practice and professional performance. A brief commentary about regulation provides an overview of professional, legal, and self-regulation expectations. This foundational ANA publication remains a key resource for nurses both to conceptualize the framework of nursing practice and to provide direction to nursing educators, administrators, and researchers. This publication also can inform other health professionals, legislators and other regulators, those who work in funding bodies, and members of the general public.

Social Context
of Nursing

"Nursing is the protection, promotion, and optimization of health and abilities, prevention of illness and injury, alleviation of suffering through the diagnosis and treatment of human response, and advocacy in the care of individuals, families, communities, and populations."

(ANA, 2003)

Nursing, like other professions, is an essential part of the society out of which it grew and within which it continues to evolve. Nursing is responsible to society in the sense that nursing's professional interest must be perceived as serving the interests of society. The mutually beneficial relationship between society and the nursing profession has been expressed as follows:

> Professions acquire recognition and relevance primarily in terms of needs, conditions, and traditions of particular societies and their members. It is societies (and often vested interests within them) that determine, in accord with their different technological and economic levels of development and their socioeconomic, political, and cultural conditions and values, what professional skills and knowledge they most need and desire. By various financial means, institutions will then emerge to train [educate] interested individuals to supply those needs.

> Logically, then, the professions open to individuals of any particular society are the property not of the individual, but of the society. What

individuals acquire through training [education] is professional knowledge and skill, not a profession or even part ownership of one. (Page, 1975, p. 7)

The Social Concerns in Health Care and Nursing

Health care continues to be a major focus of attention in the United States and worldwide. Many other societal concerns garner extensive attention and subsequent action by the nursing profession and its nurse constituency. Nursing has an active and enduring leadership role in public and political determinations about the following six key areas of health care:

- **Organization, delivery, and financing of quality health care**
  Quality health care is a human right for all (ANA, 2008b). To improve the quality of care, healthcare professionals must address these complex issues: increasing costs of care; health disparities; and the lack of safe, accessible, and available healthcare services and resources.

- **Provision for the public's health**
  Increasing responsibility for basic self-help measures by the individual, family, group, community, or population complements the use of health promotion, disease prevention, and environmental measures.

- **Expansion of nursing and healthcare knowledge and appropriate application of technology**
  Incorporation of research and evidence into practice helps inform the selection, implementation, and evaluation processes associated with the generation and application of knowledge and technology to healthcare outcomes.

- **Expansion of healthcare resources and health policy**
  Expanded facilities and workforce capacity for personal care and community health services are needed to support and enhance the capacity for self-help and self-care of individuals, families, groups, communities, and populations.

- **Definitive planning for health policy and regulation**
  Collaborative planning is responsive to consumer needs and provides for best resource use in the provision of health care for all.

- **Duties under extreme conditions**
  Health professionals will weigh their duty to provide care with obligations to their own health and that of their families during disasters, pandemics, and other extreme emergencies.

Of increasing importance, healthcare regulatory bodies set institutional standards for mandated quality of care, and other healthcare entities provide guidelines and protocols to attain quality care and better outcomes. The goals to provide quality while addressing the costs and quantity of available healthcare services will continue to be social and political priorities for nursing action.

The Authority for Nursing Practice for Nurses

The authority for nursing, as for other professions, is based on social responsibility, which in turn derives from a complex social base and a social contract.

> There is a social contract between society and the profession. Under its terms, society grants the professions authority over functions vital to itself and permits them considerable autonomy in the conduct of their own affairs. In return, the professions are expected to act responsibly, always mindful of the public trust. Self-regulation to assure quality and performance is at the heart of this relationship. It is the authentic hallmark of the mature profession. (Donabedian, 1976)

Nursing's social contract reflects the profession's long-standing core values and ethics, which provide grounding for health care in society. It is easy to overlook this social contract underlying the nursing profession when faced with certain facets of contemporary society, including depersonalization, apathy, disconnectedness, and growing globalization. But upon closer examination, we see that society validates the existence of the profession through licensure, public affirmation, and legal and legislative parameters. Nursing's response is to provide care to all who are in need, regardless of their cultural, social, or economic standing.

The nursing profession fulfills society's need for qualified and appropriately prepared individuals who embrace, and act according to, a strong code of ethics, especially when entrusted with the health care of individuals, families, groups, communities, and populations. The public ranks nurses among the top-few most trusted professionals. In turn, the nursing profession's trusted position in society imposes a responsibility to provide the very best health care. The provision of such health care relies on well-educated and clinically astute nurses and a professional association, comprising these same nurses, that establishes a code of ethics, standards of care and practice, educational and practice requirements, and policies that govern the profession.

The American Nurses Association (ANA) is the professional organization that performs an essential function in articulating, maintaining, and strengthening the social contract that exists between nursing and society, upon which the authority to practice nursing is based. That social contract is evident in ANA's most enduring and influential work, which is derived from the collective expertise of its constituent member associations, individual members, and affiliate member organizations. Such work includes:

- Developing and maintaining nursing's code of ethics;

- Developing and maintaining the scope and standards of nursing practice;

- Supporting the development of nursing theory and research to explain observations and guide nursing practice;

- Establishing the educational requirements of professional practice;

- Defining professional role competence; and

- Developing programs and resources to establish and articulate nursing's accountability to society, including practice policy work and governmental advocacy.

The Elements of Nursing's Social Contract

The following statements undergird professional nursing's social contract with society:

- Humans manifest an essential unity of mind, body, and spirit.

- Human experience is contextually and culturally defined.

- Health and illness are human experiences. The presence of illness does not preclude health, nor does optimal health preclude illness.

- The relationship between the nurse and patient occurs within the context of the values and beliefs of the patient and nurse.

- Public policy and the healthcare delivery system influence the health and well-being of society and professional nursing.

- Individual responsibility and interprofessional involvement are essential.

These values and assumptions apply whether the recipient of professional nursing care is an individual, family, group, community, or population.

Professional Collaboration in Health Care

The nursing profession is particularly focused on establishing effective working relationships and collaborative efforts essential to accomplish its health-oriented mission. Multiple factors combine to intensify the importance of direct human interactions, communication, and professional collaboration: the complexity, size, and culture of the healthcare system and its transitional and dynamic state; increasing public involvement in health policy; and a national focus on health.

Collaboration means true partnership, valuing expertise, power, and respect on all sides and recognizing and accepting separate and combined spheres of activity and responsibility. Collaboration includes mutual safeguarding of the legitimate interests of each party and a commonality of goals that is recognized by all parties. The parties base their relationship upon trust and the recognition that each one's contribution is richer and more truly real because of the strength and uniqueness of the others.

Successful collaboration requires that nursing and its members respond to diversity by recognizing, assessing, and adapting the nature of working relationships with individuals, populations, and other health professionals and health workers. These efforts also extend to relationships within nursing and between nursing and representatives of the public in all environments where nursing practice may occur.

Definition of Nursing

Definitions of nursing have evolved to reflect the essential features of professional nursing:

- Provision of a caring relationship that facilitates health and healing

- Attention to the range of human experiences and responses to health and illness within the physical and social environments

- Integration of assessment data with knowledge gained from an appreciation of the patient or the group

- Application of scientific knowledge to the processes of diagnosis and treatment through the use of judgment and critical thinking

- Advancement of professional nursing knowledge through scholarly inquiry

- Influence on social and public policy to promote social justice

- Assurance of safe, quality, and evidence-based practice

In her *Notes on Nursing: What It Is and What It Is Not*, published in 1859, Florence Nightingale defined nursing as having "charge of the personal health of somebody . . . , and what nursing has to do . . . is to put the patient in the best condition for nature to act upon him."

A century later, Virginia Henderson (1961) defined the purpose of nursing as "to assist the individual, sick or well, in the performance of those activities contributing to health or its recovery (or to a peaceful death) that he would perform unaided if he had the necessary strength, will or knowledge. And to do this in such a way as to help him gain independence as rapidly as possible."

In the original *Nursing: A Social Policy Statement* (ANA, 1980), nursing was defined as "the diagnosis and treatment of human responses to actual or potential health problems."

In 2001, ANA's *Code of Ethics With Interpretive Statements* stated that "nursing encompassed the prevention of illness, the alleviation of suffering, and the protection, promotion and restoration of health in the care of individuals, families, groups, and communities."

The definition for nursing remains unchanged from the 2003 edition of *Nursing's Social Policy Statement*:

> Nursing is the protection, promotion, and optimization of health and abilities, prevention of illness and injury, alleviation of suffering through the diagnosis and treatment of human response, and advocacy in the care of individuals, families, communities, and populations.

This definition encompasses four essential characteristics of nursing: human responses or phenomena, theory application, nursing actions or interventions, and outcomes.

Human Responses

These are the responses of individuals to actual or potential health problems, and which are the phenomena of concern to nurses. Human responses include any observable need, concern, condition, event, or fact of interest to nurses that may be the target of evidence-based nursing practice.

Theory Application

In nursing, theory is a set of interrelated concepts, definitions, or propositions used to systematically describe, explain, predict, or control human responses or phenomena of interest to nurses. Understanding theories of nursing and other disciplines precedes, and serves as a basis for, *theory application* through evidence-based nursing actions.

Nursing Actions

The aims of nursing actions (also *nursing interventions*) are to protect, promote, and optimize health; to prevent illness and injury; to alleviate suffering; and to advocate for individuals, families, communities, and populations. Nursing actions are theoretically derived, evidence-based, and require well-developed intellectual competencies.

Outcomes

The purpose of nursing actions is to produce beneficial outcomes in relation to identified human responses. Evaluation of outcomes of nursing actions determines whether the actions have been effective. Findings from nursing research provide rigorous scientific evidence of beneficial outcomes of specific nursing actions.

Figure 1 depicts the intertwined relationships of human responses, theory application, nursing actions, and outcomes.

FIGURE 1. DEFINING CHARACTERISTICS OF NURSING PRACTICE

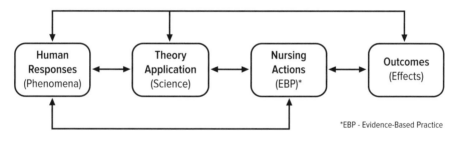

*EBP - Evidence-Based Practice

Knowledge Base for Nursing Practice

Nursing is a profession and is both a science and an art. The knowledge base for professional nursing practice includes nursing science, philosophy, and ethics; biology and psychology; and the social, physical, economic, organizational, and technological sciences. To refine and expand nursing's knowledge base, nurses use theories that fit with professional nursing's values of health and health care and that are relevant to professional nursing practice. Nurses apply research findings and implement the best evidence into their practice based on applicability to the individual, family, group, community, population, or system of care. These efforts generate knowledge and advance nursing science.

Nurses are concerned with human experiences and responses across the life span. Nurses partner with individuals, families, communities, and populations to address issues such as the following:

- Promotion of health and wellness

- Promotion of safety and quality of care

- Care, self-care processes, and care coordination

- Physical, emotional, and spiritual comfort, discomfort, and pain

- Adaptation to physiological and pathophysiological processes

- Emotions related to the experience of birth, growth and development, health, illness, disease, and death

- Meanings ascribed to health, illness, and other concepts

- Linguistic and cultural sensitivity

- Health literacy

- Decision making and the ability to make choices

- Relationships, role performance, and change processes within relationships

- Social policies and their effects on health

- Healthcare systems and their relationships to access, cost, and quality of health care

- The environment and the prevention of disease and injury

Nurses use their theoretical and evidence-based knowledge of these human experiences and responses to collaborate with patients and others to assess, diagnose, plan, implement, evaluate care, and identify outcomes. Nursing interventions aim to produce beneficial effects, contribute to quality outcomes, and—above all—do no harm. Nurses use the process that is evidence-based practice as a foundation of quality patient care to evaluate the effectiveness of care in relationship to identified outcomes.

Scope of Nursing Practice

Professional nursing has a single scope of practice that encompasses the range of activities from those of the beginning registered nurse through those of the most advanced level of nursing practice. The scope of practice statement (ANA, 2010) describes the *who, what, where, when, why*, and *how* of nursing practice. Although a single scope of professional nursing practice exists, the depth and breadth to which individual nurses engage in the total scope of professional nursing practice are dependent on their educational preparation and self-development, their experience, their role, the setting, and the nature of the populations they serve.

Further, all nurses are responsible for practicing in accordance with recognized standards of professional nursing practice and the recognized professional code of ethics. Note that the lower level and foundation of the pyramid in Figure 2 *(see next page)* includes the scope of professional practice, standards of practice, and the code of ethics.

Each nurse remains accountable for the quality of care within his or her scope of nursing practice. The level of application of standards varies with the education, experience, and skills of the individual nurse, who must rely on self-determination and self-regulation as the final level of professional accountability.

Professional nursing's scope of practice is dynamic and continually evolving, characterized by a flexible boundary responsive to the changing needs of society and the expanding knowledge base of applicable theoretical and

FIGURE 2. MODEL OF PROFESSIONAL NURSING PRACTICE

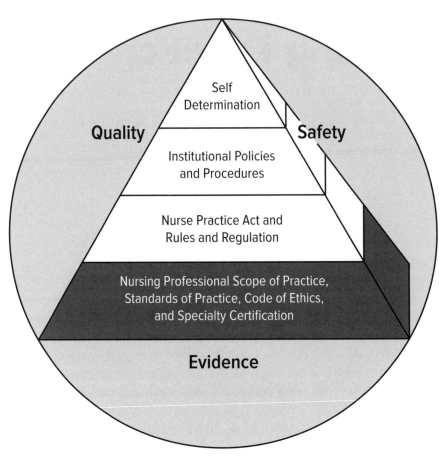

scientific domains. This scope of practice thus overlaps those of other professions involved in health care, whose boundaries are also constantly evolving. Members of any profession collaborate in various ways, such as:

- Sharing knowledge, techniques, and ideas about how to deliver and evaluate quality and outcomes in health care

- Sharing some functions and a common focus on the same overall mission

- Recognizing the expertise of others within and outside the profession, referring patients to other providers when appropriate

Nursing practice necessitates using such critical-thinking processes as the nursing process to apply the best available evidence to caregiving and promoting human functions and responses. Such caregiving includes, but is not limited to, initiating and maintaining comfort measures, establishing an environment conducive to well-being, providing health counseling, and teaching. Nurses not only independently establish plans of care but also carry out interventions prescribed by other authorized healthcare providers. Therefore, advocacy, communication, collaboration, and coordination are notable characteristics of nursing practice. Nurses base their practice on understanding the human condition across the life span and the relationship of the individual, family, group, community, or population within their own setting and environment.

Registered nurses and nurses with advanced graduate education and preparation provide and direct nursing care. All registered nurses are educated in the art and science of nursing, with the goal of helping individuals, families, groups, communities, and populations to promote, attain, maintain, and restore health or to experience dignified death. Nurses may also develop expertise in a particular specialty. The increasing complexity of care reinforces ANA's consistent advocacy (since 1965) of the baccalaureate degree in nursing as the preferred educational requirement for entry into professional nursing practice.

Specialization in Nursing Practice

Specialization involves focusing on nursing practice in a specific area, identified from within the whole field of professional nursing. ANA and specialty nursing organizations delineate the components of professional nursing practice that are essential for any particular specialty. The following characteristics must be met for ANA recognition of a nursing specialty. A nursing specialty (ANA, 2008d):

- Defines itself as nursing;

- Adheres to the overall licensure requirements of the profession;

- Subscribes to the overall purposes and functions of nursing;

- Is clearly defined;

- Can identify a need and demand for itself;

- Has a well-derived knowledge base particular to the practice of the nursing specialty;

- Is concerned with phenomena of the discipline of nursing;

- Defines competencies for the area of specialty nursing practice;

- Has existing mechanisms for supporting, reviewing, and disseminating research to support its knowledge base;

- Has defined educational criteria for specialty preparation or graduate degree;

- Has continuing education programs or continuing competence mechanisms for nurses in the specialty;

- Is organized and represented by a national or international specialty association or branch of a parent organization;

- Is practiced nationally or internationally; and

- Includes a substantial number of registered nurses who devote most of their practice to the specialty.

Registered nurses may seek certification in a variety of specialized areas of nursing practice as a demonstration of competence (ANA, 2008c).

Advanced Nursing Practice

Advanced nursing practice builds on the competencies of the registered nurse and is characterized by the integration and application of a broad range of theoretical and evidence-based knowledge that occurs as part of graduate nursing education.

Advanced Practice Registered Nurses

Advanced practice registered nurses (APRNs) hold master's or doctoral degrees in nursing, are certified in their designated specialty practice areas, and are recognized and approved to practice in their roles by state boards of nursing or other regulatory oversight bodies, often through special professional licensing processes.

APRNs are educationally prepared in one of the four APRN roles (certified nurse practitioners, certified registered nurse anesthetists, certified nurse-midwives, and clinical nurse specialists) and in at least one of six possible population foci: family/individual across the life span; adult/gerontology; neonatal;

pediatrics; women's health/gender-related health; psychiatric/mental health). Education, certification, and licensure of these individuals should be congruent with role and population foci (APRN Consensus, 2008). APRN specialty practice may focus on specific populations beyond those identified or focus on healthcare needs (such as oncology, palliative care, substance abuse, nephrology) that meet criteria for specialization as identified in the APRN Consensus Model. (See Appendix A for the full text of the APRN Consensus Model.)

Additional Specialized Advanced Nursing Positions

The profession of nursing is also dependent on continued expansion of nursing knowledge, education of nurses, appropriate organization and administration of nursing services, and development and adoption of policies consistent with values and assumptions that underlie the scope of professional nursing practice. Registered nurses may practice in such advanced positions as nurse educator, nurse administrator, nurse researcher, nurse policy analyst, advanced public health nurse, and informatics nurse specialist. These advanced roles require specific additional knowledge and skills gained through graduate-level education, holding master's or doctoral degrees.

Further details on the scope of professional nursing practice and the specifics that describe the *who, what, where, when, why,* and *how* of nursing practice for all registered nurses appear in the current version of *Nursing: Scope and Standards of Practice* (ANA, 2010).

Standards of Professional Nursing Practice

To guide professional practice, nursing has established standards of professional nursing practice, which are further categorized into standards of practice and standards of professional performance.

Definition and Function of Standards

Standards are authoritative statements by which the nursing profession describes the responsibilities for which its practitioners are accountable. Standards reflect the values and priorities of the profession and provide direction for professional nursing practice and a framework for the evaluation of this practice. They also define the nursing profession's accountability to the public and the outcomes for which registered nurses are responsible (ANA, 2010).

Development of Standards

A professional nursing organization has a responsibility to its members and to the public it serves to develop standards of practice and standards of professional performance that may pertain to general or specialty practice. The American Nurses Association, as the professional organization for all registered nurses, has assumed the responsibility for developing generic standards that apply to the practice of all professional nurses. However, standards belong to the profession and thus require broad input into their development and revision. The scope and standards of practice developed by ANA describe a competent level of nursing practice and professional performance common to all registered nurses (ANA, 2010).

Standards of Professional Nursing Practice

The Standards of Professional Nursing Practice are comprised of the Standards of Practice and the Standards of Professional Performance.

Standards of Practice

The Standards of Practice describe a competent level of nursing care, as demonstrated by the critical thinking model known as the *nursing process*, which includes the components of assessment, diagnosis, outcomes identification, planning, implementation, and evaluation. These standards encompass significant actions taken by registered nurses and form the foundation of the nurse's decision making.

Standards of Professional Performance

The Standards of Professional Performance describe a competent level of behavior in the professional role, including activities related to quality of practice, education, professional practice evaluation, collegiality, collaboration, ethics, research, resource utilization, and leadership. Registered nurses are accountable for their professional actions to themselves, their patients, their peers, and ultimately to society.

The nursing process is usually conceptualized and presented as the integration of singular, concurrent actions of assessment, diagnosis, identification of outcomes, planning, implementation, and, finally, evaluation. Most often the nursing process is introduced to nursing students as a linear process with a feedback loop from evaluation to assessment, as reflected in Figure 3.

Figure 4 reflects how the nursing process in practice is not linear, but relies heavily on the bidirectional feedback loops from and to each component. The standards of practice are co-located near the steps of the nursing process to represent the directive nature of the standards as the professional nurse completes each component of the nursing process. Similarly, the standards of professional performance relate to how the professional nurse adheres to the standards of practice, completes the nursing process, and addresses other nursing practice issues and concerns.

FIGURE 3. THE NURSING PROCESS

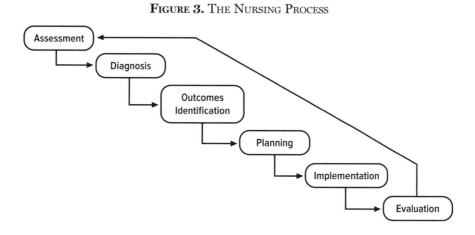

FIGURE 4. THE NURSING PROCESS AND THE STANDARDS
OF PROFESSIONAL NURSING PRACTICE

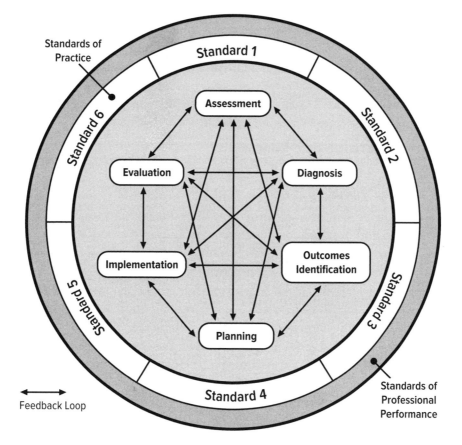

Application of Scope and Standards

Content within the current edition of *Nursing: Scope and Standards of Practice* should serve as the basis for the following:

- Policies, procedures, and protocols

- Position descriptions and performance appraisals

- Certification activities

- Educational programs and offerings

- Development and evaluation of nursing service delivery systems and organizational structures, including the application of technologies

- Specialty nursing scope and standards of practice

- Quality improvement systems

- Databases

- Regulatory systems

- Healthcare reimbursement and financing methodologies

- Establishing the legal standard of care

Code of Ethics for Nurses

The current code of ethics for the profession, *Code of Ethics for Nurses With Interpretive Statements* (ANA, 2001) "functions as a general guide for the profession's members and as a social contract with the public that it serves" (Fowler, 2008, p. xi). It is the profession's expression of the values, duties, and commitments to that public. Its nine provisions give voice to professional nurses and delineate what the nurse owes not only to others but also to him- or herself. This includes, but is not limited to, personal and professional growth, preserving integrity, and safety (Fowler, 2008).

Although the Code of Ethics for Nurses is intended to be a living document for nurses, and health care is becoming more complex, the basic tenets found within this particular code of ethics remain unchanged. For example, *Guide to the Code of Ethics for Nurses: Interpretation and Application* (Fowler, 2008) provides interpretation and examples of the application of the nine ethical provisions.

Autonomy and Competent Practice

Autonomy is the capacity of a nurse to determine his or her own actions through independent choice within the full scope of nursing practice (Ballou, 1998). Competence is foundational to autonomy: the public has a right to expect nurses to demonstrate professional competence. The nursing profession and professional associations must shape and guide any practice, assuring nursing competence.

The key indicators of competent practice are identified with each standard of practice and professional performance. For a standard to be met, all the listed competencies must be met. An individual who demonstrates competence is performing successfully at an expected level. A *competency* is an expected level of performance that integrates knowledge, skills, abilities, and judgment. Standards should remain stable over time because they reflect the philosophical values of the profession. Competency statements, however, may be revised more frequently to incorporate advances in scientific knowledge and expectations for nursing practice.

Assurance of competence is the shared responsibility of the profession, individual nurses, professional organizations, credentialing and certification entities, regulatory agencies, employers, and other key stakeholders (ANA, 2008c).

Regulation of Professional Nursing

Figure 5 *(see next page)* depicts the roles and relationships associated with the regulation of nursing practice. The model recognizes the contributions of professional and specialty nursing organizations, educational institutions, credentialing and accrediting organizations, and regulatory agencies; explains the role of workplace policies and procedures; and confirms the individual nurse's ultimate responsibility and accountability for defining nursing practice (Styles, Schumann, Bickford, & White, 2008).

The Scope of Nursing Practice, the Standards of Professional Nursing Practice, and the Code of Ethics for Nurses serve as the foundation for legislation and regulatory policies to assure protection of the public's safety (Styles, Schumann, Bickford, & White, 2008).

Under the terms of a social contract between society and the profession, society grants authority over functions vital to the profession and permits considerable autonomy in the conduct of its own affairs. Professional nursing, like other professions, is accountable for ensuring that its members act in the public interest while providing the unique service that society has entrusted to them. The processes by which the profession does this include professional regulation, legal regulation, and self-regulation. The Scope of Nursing Practice, the Standards of Professional Nursing Practice, the Code of Ethics for Nurses, and the current social policy statement are components of professional regulation and serve as the foundation for legislation, regulatory policy making, and nursing practice that may be set in place to help assure protection of the public's safety.

FIGURE 5. MODEL OF PROFESSIONAL NURSING PRACTICE REGULATION

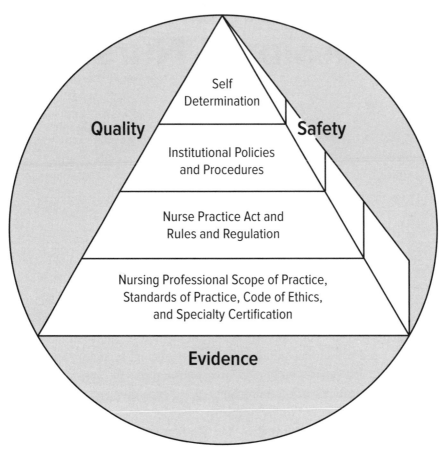

Professional Regulation

Professional regulation is a profession's oversight, monitoring, and control of its members based on principles, guidelines, and rules deemed important. Professional regulation of nursing practice begins with the professional definition of nursing and the delineation of the scope of professional nursing practice. Professional standards are derived from the scope of nursing practice.

The social contract for nursing has been made specific through the professional society's work, derived from the collective expertise of the American Nurses Association, in collaboration with members of its constituent member associations and members of other nursing organizations. These responsibilities include the following:

- Establishing and maintaining a professional code of ethics

- Determining standards of practice

- Fostering the development of nursing theory, derived from nursing research

- Establishing nursing practice built on a base of best evidence

- Establishing the specifications for the educational requirements for entry into professional practice at basic and advanced levels

- Developing certification processes as measures of professional competence

Certification is a judgment of competence made by nurses who are themselves practicing within the area of specialization. Certification is the formal recognition of the knowledge, skills, abilities, judgment, and experience demonstrated by the achievement of formal criteria identified by the profession. Credentialing boards develop and implement certification examinations and procedures for nurses who wish to have their specialty-practice knowledge recognized by the profession and the public. One component of the required evidence is successful completion of an examination that tests the knowledge base for the selected area of practice. Other requirements relate to the requisite content of course work and the amount of practice hours. Credentialing bodies may elect to use professional portfolios as psychometrically and legally defensible alternatives for certification examinations. Professional portfolios provide a comprehensive and reflective representation of professional abilities, achievements, and efforts.

Contemporary specialty nursing practice is in transition in response to the increasing complexity of care and exponential explosion of data, information, and knowledge. Specialization is a mark of the advancement of the nursing profession and assists in clarifying, revising, and strengthening existing practice. Specialization not only expedites the production of new knowledge and its application in practice, but also provides preparation for teaching and research related to any defined area of nursing. The specialist in nursing practice is evolving to be a nurse who has become expert in a defined area of knowledge and nursing practice through study and supervised practice at the graduate (master's or doctoral) level.

Legal Regulation

Legal regulation is the oversight, monitoring, and control of designated professionals, based on applicable statutes and regulations, accompanied by the interpretation of these laws. All nurses are legally accountable for actions taken in the course of professional nursing practice, as well as for actions delegated by the nurse to others assisting in provision of nursing care. Such accountability is accomplished through legal regulatory mechanisms of licensure; granting of authority to practice, such as nurse practice acts; and criminal and civil laws.

The legal contract between society and the professions is defined by statute and by associated rules and regulations. State nurse practice acts and related legislation and regulations serve as the explicit codification of the profession's obligation to act in the best interests of society. Nurse practice acts grant nurses the authority to practice and grant society the authority to sanction nurses who violate the norms of the profession or act in a manner that threatens the safety of the public.

Statutory definitions of nursing should be compatible with, and build upon, the profession's definition of its practice base. They must be general enough to provide for the dynamic nature of an evolving scope of nursing practice. Society is best served when consistent definitions of the scope of nursing and of advanced practice nursing are used by each state's board of nursing and other regulatory bodies. This allows residents of all states to access the full range of nursing services. Multiple stakeholders have established a collaborative effort to garner consensus in this arena.

Institutional Policies and Procedures

Nursing practice occurs within societal institutions, organizations, and settings that have accompanying policies, procedures, rules, and regulations. The scope and standards of practice for nursing and nursing specialties should help guide development of institutional policies and procedures to create a more detailed representation of what constitutes safe, quality, and evidence-based nursing practice.

Self-Regulation

Self-regulation, which requires personal accountability for the knowledge base for professional practice, is an individual's demonstrated personal control based on principles, guidelines, and rules deemed important. Nurses develop

FIGURE **6.** SELF-DETERMINATION IN THE MODEL OF
PROFESSIONAL NURSING PRACTICE REGULATION

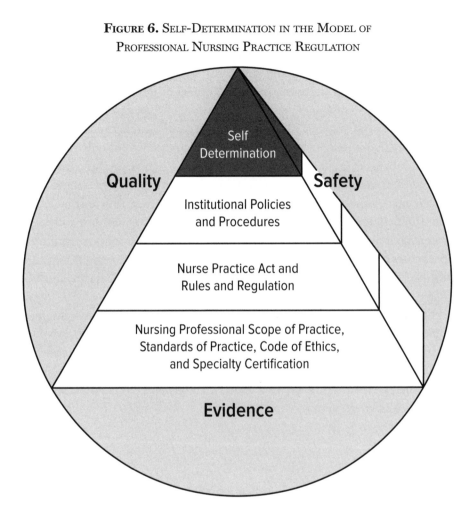

and maintain current knowledge, skills, and abilities through formal academic programs and continuing education professional development programs. When available, nurses pursue certification in their area of practice to demonstrate this competence.

Nurses exercise autonomy and freedom within their scope of practice. Autonomy is defined as the capacity of a nurse to determine his or her own actions through independent choice within the full scope of nursing practice (Ballou, 1998). Autonomy and freedom are based on the nurse's commitment to self-regulation and accountability for practice. In Figure 6, the apex of the pyramid, labeled Self-Determination, represents autonomy, self-regulation, and accountability for practice.

Competence is foundational to autonomy. Nursing competency is an expected level of performance that integrates knowledge, skills, abilities, and judgment (ANA, 2008d). Greater autonomy and freedom in nursing practice are based on broader authority rooted in expert or advanced knowledge in selected areas of nursing. This expert knowledge is associated with greater self-discipline and responsibility for direct care practice and for advancement of the nursing profession. A greater degree of autonomy not only imposes a greater duty to act and to do so competently but also increases accountability.

Nurses also regulate their own practice by participating in peer review. Continuous performance improvement fosters the refinement of knowledge, skills, and clinical decision-making processes at all levels and in all areas of professional nursing practice. As expressed in the profession's code of ethics, peer review is one mechanism by which nurses are held accountable for practice. As noted in Provision 3.4 (Standards and Review Mechanism) in *Code of Ethics for Nurses with Interpretive Statements*, nurses should also be active participants in the development of policies and review mechanisms designed to promote patient safety, reduce the likelihood of errors, and address both environmental system factors and human factors that present increased risk to patients. In addition, when errors do occur, nurses are expected to follow established guidelines in reporting committed or observed errors. The focus should be directed to improving systems, rather than projecting blame.

Application of Nursing's Social Policy Statement

Registered nurses should find the content within *Nursing's Social Policy Statement: The Essence of the Profession* pertinent to everyday practice. The description of nursing as a profession valued within society, definition of nursing, presentation of the nursing process, and discussion of regulation set the stage for practice by promoting understanding.

Nursing faculty should find content within this edition of *Nursing's Social Policy Statement* that is critical for inclusion in curricula and course materials in undergraduate-, graduate-, and doctoral-level education. Similarly, nurses in professional development roles reinforce the concepts presented in this resource in the practice setting, especially those related to autonomy, competence, scope and standards of nursing practice, and the nursing process.

Students will benefit from reading this statement on nursing's social policy as they learn about the evolution of their profession through its key attributes: the definition of nursing, the profession's delineation of the characteristics of a nursing specialty, and the delineation of its scope of practice and accompanying standards and competency statements. The models depicting the nursing process, with its feedback loops and the relationship of the standards of practice and professional performance to the nursing process, will be invaluable in generating improved understanding of the complexity of nursing practice.

Similarly, clear delineation of the six social concerns in health care, and other statements that undergird nursing's social contract with society, reaffirm the importance of collaboration within nursing and interprofessional healthcare teams. Registered nurses will experience even greater relevance of this content in every practice setting.

Nurse administrators should use this nursing social policy statement as a resource for strategic planning activities, public explanations about nursing and its registered nurses, and the development of vision and mission statements. Members of legal and regulatory bodies and organizations should review this document to understand better how professional, self-, and legal regulation can complement—rather than conflict with—each other. Healthcare consumers may wish to use the social policy statement to understand better the foundation upon which the nursing profession and its registered nurses base their practice.

Conclusion

This social policy statement describes the pivotal nature and role of professional nursing in society and health care. The definition of nursing, introduction of the scope and accompanying standards of professional nursing practice, and discussion of specialization and regulation within the social context in which nurses practice provide an overview of the essence of nursing. Registered nurses focus their specialized knowledge, skills, and caring on improving the health status of the public and ensuring safe, effective, quality care. This statement serves as a resource to assist nurses in conceptualizing their professional practice and provides direction to educators, administrators, and researchers within nursing. This statement also informs other health professionals, legislators and other regulators, funding bodies, and the public about nursing's social responsibility, accountability, and contribution to health care.

References

All web-based references were retrieved May 31, 2010.

American Nurses Association. (1980). *Nursing: A social policy statement.* Kansas City, MO: American Nurses Publishing.

American Nurses Association. (2001). *Code of ethics for nurses with interpretive statements.* Silver Spring, MD: Nursesbooks.org.

American Nurses Association. (2002). *Nursing's agenda for the future: A call to the nation.* http://nursingworld.org/MainMenuCategories/ HealthcareandPolicyIssues/Reports.aspx

American Nurses Association. (2003). *Nursing's social policy statement* (2nd ed.). Silver Spring, MD: Nursesbooks.org.

American Nurses Association. (2010). *Nursing: Scope and standards of practice* (2nd ed.). Silver Spring, MD: Nursesbooks.org.

American Nurses Association. (2008a). *Adapting standards of care under extreme conditions: Guidance for professionals during disasters, pandemics, and other extreme emergencies.* Silver Spring, MD: Author.

American Nurses Association. (2008b). *ANA's health system reform agenda.* www.nursingworld.org/healthreformagenda

American Nurses Association. (2008c). *Professional role competence position statement.* http://nursingworld.org/MainMenuCategories/ HealthcareandPolicyIssues/ANAPositionStatements/practice/ PositionStatementProfessionalRoleCompetence.aspx

American Nurses Association. (2008d). *Recognition of a nursing specialty, approval of a specialty nursing scope of practice statement, and acknowledgment of specialty nursing standards of practice.* Silver Spring, MD: Author.

APRN Consensus Work Group & National Council of State Boards of Nursing APRN Advisory Committee. (2008). *Consensus model for APRN regulation: Licensure, accreditation, certification and education.* http:// www.nursingworld.org/ConsensusModelforAPRN

Ballou, K. A. (1998). Concept analysis of autonomy. *Journal of Professional Nursing,* 14(2), 102–110.

Donabedian, A. (1976). Forward, in M. Phaneuf, *The nursing audit: Self-regulation in nursing practice* (2nd ed., p. 8). New York: Appleton-Century-Crofts.

Fowler, Marsha D. M. (Ed.). (2008). *Guide to the code of ethics for nurses: Interpretation and application.* Silver Spring, MD: Nursesbooks.org.

Henderson, V. (1961). *Basic principles of nursing care* (p. 42). London: International Council of Nurses.

Nightingale, F. (1859). *Notes on nursing: What it is and what it is not* (Preface, p. 75). London: Harrison and Sons. (Facsimile ed., J. B. Lippincott Company, 1946).

Page, B. B. (1975). Who owns the profession? *Hastings Center Report, 5* (5, October), 7–8. The Hastings Center: Garrison, NY.

Styles, M. M., Schumann, M. J., Bickford, C. J., & White, K. M. (2008). *Specialization and credentialing in nursing revisited: Understanding the issues, advancing the profession.* Silver Spring, MD: Nursesbooks.org.

Glossary

Advanced practice registered nurse (APRN) A certified nurse practitioner, certified registered nurse anesthetist, certified nurse midwife, or clinical nurse specialist who is educationally prepared (usually at a post-baccalaureate level), accredited by a national accrediting body, and has current certification by a national certifying body in the appropriate APRN role and at least one population focus. *See also* Population focus; *each type of APRN.*

Autonomy The capacity of a nurse to determine his/her own actions through independent choice, including demonstration of competence, within the full scope of nursing practice.

Certified nurse practitioner (CNP) A registered nurse who is professionally prepared to provide direct primary care and acute care (initial, ongoing, and comprehensive) along the wellness–illness continuum and in all settings. Clinical CNP care includes health promotion, disease prevention, health education, and counseling as well as the diagnosis and management of acute and chronic diseases (APRN Consensus, 2008).

Certified registered nurse anesthetist (CRNA) A registered nurse who is prepared to provide full-spectrum anesthesia care and anesthesia-related care for individuals across the lifespan, whose health status may range from healthy through all recognized levels of acuity, including persons with immediate, severe, or life-threatening illnesses or injury (APRN Consensus, 2008).

Certified nurse midwife (CNM) A registered nurse who is prepared to provide primary health care services to women throughout the lifespan, including gynecologic care, family planning services, preconception care, prenatal and postpartum care, childbirth, care of the newborn, and treating the male partner of the female client for sexually transmitted disease and reproductive health (APRN Consensus, 2008).

Clinical nurse specialist (CNS) A registered nurse who is professionally prepared to integrate care across the continuum and through the patient, nurse, and system spheres of influence. The primary CNS goal is continuous improvement of patient outcomes and nursing care. The CNS is responsible and accountable for diagnosis and treatment of health/illness states, disease management, health promotion, and prevention of illness and risk behaviors (APRN Consensus, 2008).

Code of ethics (nursing) A set of provisions that makes explicit the primary goals, values, and obligations of the nursing profession and expresses its values, duties, and commitments to the society of which it is a part. In the United States, nurses abide by and adhere to the Code of Ethics for Nurses (ANA, 2001).

Collaboration A professional healthcare partnership grounded in a reciprocal and respectful recognition and acceptance of each partner's unique expertise, power, and sphere of influence and responsibilities; the commonality of goals; the mutual safeguarding of the legitimate interest of each party; and the advantages of such a relationship.

Competency An expected and measurable level of nursing performance that integrates knowledge, skills, abilities, and judgment that is based on established scientific knowledge and expectations for nursing practice.

Evidence-based practice A scholarly and systematic problem-solving paradigm that results in the delivery of high quality health care.

Human responses The phenomena of concern to nurses that include any observable need, concern, condition, event, or fact of interest actual or potential health problems.

Nursing The protection, promotion, and optimization of health and abilities, prevention of illness and injury, alleviation of suffering through the diagnosis and treatment of human response, and advocacy in the care of individuals, families, communities, and populations.

Nursing actions Theoretically derived and evidence-based interventions that are intended to protect, promote, and optimize health; prevent illness and injury; alleviate suffering; advocate for individuals, families, communities, and populations; and otherwise produce beneficial outcomes.

Nursing practice The collective professional activities of nurses that are characterized by the interrelations of human responses, theory application, nursing actions, and outcomes.

Nursing process A critical thinking model comprising the integration of singular, concurrent actions of these six components: assessment, diagnosis, identification of outcomes, planning, implementation, and evaluation.

Outcomes (nursing) The results of nursing actions, in relation to identified human responses, based on findings from nursing research, the efficacy and benefit of which are determined by evaluation.

Population focus Any one of these six APRN practice areas: family/individual across the life span; adult/gerontology; neonatal; pediatrics; women's health/gender-related health; psychiatric/mental health.

Registered nurse (RN) An individual registered or licensed by a state, commonwealth, territory, government, or other regulatory body to practice as a registered nurse.

Regulation of nursing practice The processes of governance and controls established by authorized bodies as standards, guidelines, protocols, and other mandates for defining, attaining, and maintaining mandated quality of care and practice.

Scope of Nursing Practice The description of the *who, what, where, when, why,* and *how* of nursing practice that addresses the range of nursing practice activities common to all registered nurses. When considered in conjunction with the Standards of Professional Nursing Practice and the Code of Ethics for Nurses, the competent level of nursing common to all registered nurses is comprehensively described.

Standards (nursing) Authoritative statements by which the nursing profession describes the responsibilities for which its practitioners are accountable, the outcomes for which registered nurses are responsible, and by which the quality of practice, service, or education can be evaluated.

Standards of Practice The subset of nursing standards that describes a competent level of nursing care as demonstrated by the nursing process that forms the basis for the decision making of registered nurses and that encompasses all significant nursing actions. *See also:* Nursing process.

Standards of Professional Nursing Practice The set of nursing standards comprised of the Standards of Practice and the Standards of Professional Performance, with each constituent standard having its own set of key indicators of competence. For a standard to be met, all the listed competencies must be met. When considered in conjunction with the Scope of Nursing Practice, comprehensively describes the competent level of nursing common to all registered nurses.

Standards of Professional Performance The subset of nursing standards that describes a competent level of activities and behavior in the professional role for the registered nurse by which they are accountable for their professional actions to themselves, their patients, their peers, and society.

Theory (nursing) A set of interrelated concepts, definitions, or propositions used to systematically describe, explain, predict, or control human responses or phenomena of interest to nurses.

Appendix A.

Consensus Model for APRN Regulation: Licensure, Accreditation, Certification and Education (2008)

The content in this appendix is not current and is of historical significance only.

Consensus Model for APRN Regulation:
Licensure, Accreditation, Certification & Education

July 7, 2008

Completed through the work of the APRN Consensus Work Group & the
National Council of State Boards of Nursing APRN Advisory Committee

About the Consensus Model Report

As underscored by the inclusion of APRNs in recent health system reform efforts, there is increased appreciation of the important role that APRNs can play in improving access to quality cost-effective care. However, a proliferation of nursing specializations, debates on appropriate credentials and scope of practice, and a lack of uniformity in state regulations have limited the ability of patients to access APRN care.

The document that is reproduced in this appendix, and that was completed in July 2008 and endorsed by 44 organizations, delineates the model for future regulation of advanced practice registered nurses. This Consensus Model, when implemented, will standardize each aspect of the regulatory process for APRNs, resulting in increased mobility for APRNs and increased access to APRN care.

The document was completed through the collaborative work of the APRN Consensus Workgroup and National Council of State Boards of Nursing APRN Advisory Committee, with extensive input from the larger APRN stakeholder community.

(SOURCE: American Nurses Association, 2009: http://www.nursingworld.org/cmissuebrief)

**Consensus Model for APRN Regulation:
Licensure, Accreditation, Certification & Education**

July 7, 2008

**Completed through the work of the APRN Consensus Work Group & the
National Council of State Boards of Nursing APRN Advisory Committee**

APRN Joint Dialogue Group Report, July 7, 2008

The APRN Consensus Work Group and the APRN Joint Dialogue Group members would like to recognize the significant contribution to the development of this report made by Jean Johnson, PhD, RN-C, FAAN, Senior Associate Dean, Health Sciences, George Washington School of Medicine and Health Sciences. Consensus could not have been reached without her experienced and dedicated facilitation of these two national, multi-organizational groups.

2

APRN Joint Dialogue Group Report, July 7, 2008

LIST OF ENDORSING ORGANIZATIONS

This Final Report of the APRN Consensus Work Group and the National Council of State Boards of Nursing APRN Advisory Committee has been disseminated to participating organizations. The names of endorsing organizations will be added periodically.

The following organizations have endorsed the Consensus Model for APRN Regulation: Licensure, Accreditation, Certification, and Education:

(Posted July 2009)
N=46

Academy of Medical-Surgical Nurses (AMSN)
Accreditation Commission for Midwifery Education (ACME)
American Academy of Nurse Practitioners (AANP)
American Academy of Nurse Practitioners Certification Program
American Association of Colleges of Nursing (AACN)
American Association of Critical-Care Nurses (AACN)
American Association of Critical-Care Nurses Certification Corporation
American Association of Legal Nurse Consultants (AALNC)
American Association of Nurse Anesthetists (AANA)
American Board of Nursing Specialties (ABNS)
American College of Nurse-Midwives (ACNM)
American College of Nurse Practitioners (ACNP)
American Holistic Nurses Association (AHNA)
American Midwifery Certification Board (AMCB)
American Nurses Association (ANA)
American Nurses Credentialing Center (ANCC)
American Psychiatric Nurses Association (APNA)
Arkansas State Board of Nursing
Association of Faculties of Pediatric Nurse Practitioners (AFPNP)
Commission on Collegiate Nursing Education (CCNE)
Council on Accreditation of Nurse Anesthesia Educational Programs (COA)
Dermatology Nurses Association (DNA)
Dermatology Nursing Certification Board (DNCB)
Emergency Nurses Association (ENA)
Gerontological Advanced Practice Nurses Association (GAPNA)
Hospice and Palliative Nurses Association (HPNA)
The International Society of Psychiatric Nurses (ISPN)
National Association of Clinical Nurse Specialists (NACNS)
National Association of Orthopedic Nurses (NAON)
National Association of Pediatric Nurse Practitioners (NAPNAP)
National Board for Certification of Hospice and Palliative Nurses (NBCHPN)
National Board on Certification & Recertification of Nurse Anesthetists (NBCRNA)
National Certification Corporation (NCC)
National Council of State Boards of Nursing (NCSBN)
National Gerontological Nursing Association (NGNA)
National League for Nursing (NLN)

3

APRN Joint Dialogue Group Report, July 7, 2008

National League for Nursing Accrediting Commission, Inc. (NLNAC)
National Organization of Nurse Practitioner Faculties (NONPF)
Nurse Practitioners in Women's Health (NPWH)
Nurses Organization of Veterans Affairs (NOVA)
Oncology Nursing Certification Corporation (ONCC)
Oncology Nursing Society (ONS)
Orthopedic Nurses Certification Board (ONCB)
Pediatric Nursing Certification Board (PNCB)
Wound, Ostomy and Continence Nurses Society (WOCN)
Wound, Ostomy and Continence Nursing Certification Board (WOCNCB)

4

APRN Joint Dialogue Group Report, July 7, 2008

INTRODUCTION

Advanced Practice Registered Nurses (APRNs) have expanded in numbers and capabilities over the past several decades with APRNs being highly valued and an integral part of the health care system. Because of the importance of APRNs in caring for the current and future health needs of patients, the education, accreditation, certification and licensure of APRNs need to be effectively aligned in order to continue to ensure patient safety while expanding patient access to APRNs.

APRNs include certified registered nurse anesthetists, certified nurse-midwives, clinical nurse specialists and certified nurse practitioners. Each has a unique history and context, but shares the commonality of being APRNs. While education, accreditation, and certification are necessary components of an overall approach to preparing an APRN for practice, the licensing boards-governed by state regulations and statutes-are the final arbiters of who is recognized to practice within a given state. Currently, there is no uniform model of regulation of APRNs across the states. Each state independently determines the APRN legal scope of practice, the roles that are recognized, the criteria for entry-into advanced practice and the certification examinations accepted for entry-level competence assessment. This has created a significant barrier for APRNs to easily move from state to state and has decreased access to care for patients.

Many nurses with advanced graduate nursing preparation practice in roles and specialties e.g., informatics, public health, education, or administration) that are essential to advance the health of the public but do not focus on direct care to individuals and, therefore, their practice does not require regulatory recognition beyond the Registered Nurse license granted by state boards of nursing. Like the four current APRN roles, practice in these other advanced specialty nursing roles requires specialized knowledge and skills acquired through graduate-level education. Although extremely important to the nursing profession and to the delivery of safe, high quality patient care, these other advanced, graduate nursing roles, which do not focus on direct patient care, are not roles for Advanced Practice Registered Nurses (APRN) and are not the subject or focus of the Regulatory Model presented in this paper.

The model for APRN regulation is the product of substantial work conducted by the Advanced Practice Nursing Consensus Work Group and the National Council of State Boards of Nursing (NCSBN) APRN Committee. While these groups began work independent of each other, they came together through representatives of each group participating in what was labeled the APRN Joint Dialogue Group. The outcome of this work has been unanimous agreement on most of the recommendations included in this document. In a few instances, when agreement was not unanimous a 66% majority was used to determine the final recommendation. However, extensive dialogue and transparency in the decision-making process is reflected in each recommendation. The background of each group can be found on pages 13-16 and individual and organizational participants in each group in Appendices C-H.

This document defines APRN practice, describes the APRN regulatory model, identifies the titles to be used, defines specialty, describes the emergence of new roles and population foci, and presents strategies for implementation.

5

APRN Joint Dialogue Group Report, July 7, 2008

Overview of APRN Model of Regulation

The APRN Model of Regulation described will be the model of the future. It is recognized that current regulation of APRNs does not reflect all of the components described in this paper and will evolve incrementally over time. A proposed timeline for implementation is presented at the end of the paper.

In this APRN model of regulation there are four roles: certified registered nurse anesthetist (CRNA), certified nurse-midwife (CNM), clinical nurse specialist (CNS), and certified nurse practitioner (CNP). These four roles are given the title of advanced practice registered nurse (APRN). APRNs are educated in one of the four roles and in at least one of six population foci: family/individual across the lifespan, adult-gerontology, pediatrics, neonatal, women's health/gender-related or psych/mental health. APRN education programs, including degree-granting and post-graduate education programs[1], are accredited. APRN education consists of a broad-based education, including three separate graduate-level courses in advanced physiology/pathophysiology, health assessment and pharmacology as well as appropriate clinical experiences. All developing APRN education programs or tracks go through a pre-approval, pre-accreditation, or accreditation process prior to admitting students. APRN education programs must be housed within graduate programs that are nationally accredited[2] and their graduates must be eligible for national certification used for state licensure.

Individuals who have the appropriate education will sit for a certification examination to assess national competencies of the APRN core, role and at least one population focus area of practice for regulatory purposes. APRN certification programs will be accredited by a national certification accrediting body[3]. APRN certification programs will require a continued competency mechanism.

Individuals will be licensed as independent practitioners for practice at the level of one of the four APRN roles within at least one of the six identified population foci. Education, certification, and licensure of an individual must be congruent in terms of role and population foci. APRNs may specialize but they cannot be licensed solely within a specialty area. *In addition, specialties can provide depth in one's practice within the established population foci*. Education and assessment strategies for specialty areas will be developed by the nursing profession, i.e., nursing organizations and special interest groups. Education for a specialty can occur concurrently with APRN education required for licensure or through post-graduate education. Competence at the specialty level will not be assessed or regulated by boards of nursing but rather by the professional organizations.

---

[1] Degree granting programs include master's and doctoral programs. Post-graduate programs include both post-master's and post-doctoral certificate education programs.
[2] APRN education programs must be accredited by a nursing accrediting organization that is recognized by the U.S. Department of Education (USDE) and/or the Council for Higher Education Accreditation (CHEA), including the Commission on Collegiate Nursing Education (CCNE), National League for Nursing Accrediting Commission (NLNAC), Council on Accreditation of Nurse Anesthesia Educational Programs (COA), Accreditation Commission for Midwifery Education (ACME), and the National Association of Nurse Practitioners in Women's Health Council on Accreditation.
[3] The certification program should be nationally accredited by the American Board of Nursing Specialties (ABNS) or the National Commission for Certifying Agencies (NCCA).

6

APRN Joint Dialogue Group Report, July 7, 2008

In addition, a mechanism that enhances the communication and transparency among APRN licensure, accreditation, certification and education bodies (LACE) will be developed and supported.

APRN REGULATORY MODEL

APRN Regulation includes the essential elements: licensure, accreditation, certification and education (LACE).

- Licensure is the granting of authority to practice.
- Accreditation is the formal review and approval by a recognized agency of educational degree or certification programs in nursing or nursing-related programs.
- Certification is the formal recognition of the knowledge, skills, and experience demonstrated by the achievement of standards identified by the profession.
- Education is the formal preparation of APRNs in graduate degree-granting or post-graduate certificate programs.

The APRN Regulatory Model applies to all elements of LACE. Each of these elements plays an essential part in the implementation of the model.

Definition of Advanced Practice Registered Nurse
Characteristics of the advanced practice registered nurse (APRN) were identified and several definitions of an APRN were considered, including the NCSBN and the American Nurses Association (ANA) definitions, as well as others. The characteristics identified aligned closely with these existing definitions. The definition of an APRN, delineated in this document, includes language that addresses responsibility and accountability for health promotion and the assessment, diagnosis, and management of patient problems, which includes the use and prescription of pharmacologic and non-pharmacologic interventions.

The definition of an Advanced Practice Registered Nurse (APRN) is a nurse:
1. who has completed an accredited graduate-level education program preparing him/her for one of the four recognized APRN roles;
2. who has passed a national certification examination that measures APRN, role and population-focused competencies and who maintains continued competence as evidenced by recertification in the role and population through the national certification program;
3. who has acquired advanced clinical knowledge and skills preparing him/her to provide direct care to patients, as well as a component of indirect care; however, the defining factor for **all** APRNs is that a significant component of the education and practice focuses on direct care of individuals;
4. whose practice builds on the competencies of registered nurses (RNs) by demonstrating a greater depth and breadth of knowledge, a greater synthesis of data, increased complexity of skills and interventions, and greater role autonomy;
5. who is educationally prepared to assume responsibility and accountability for health promotion and/or maintenance as well as the assessment, diagnosis, and management of patient problems, which includes the use and prescription of pharmacologic and non-pharmacologic interventions;
6. who has clinical experience of sufficient depth and breadth to reflect the intended license; **and**

7

APRN Joint Dialogue Group Report, July 7, 2008

7. who has obtained a license to practice as an APRN in one of the four APRN roles: certified registered nurse anesthetist (CRNA), certified nurse-midwife (CNM), clinical nurse specialist (CNS), or certified nurse practitioner (CNP).

Advanced practice registered nurses are licensed independent practitioners who are expected to practice within standards established or recognized by a licensing body. Each APRN is accountable to patients, the nursing profession, and the licensing board to comply with the requirements of the state nurse practice act and the quality of advanced nursing care rendered; for recognizing limits of knowledge and experience, planning for the management of situations beyond the APRN's expertise; and for consulting with or referring patients to other health care providers as appropriate.

All APRNs are educationally prepared to provide a scope of services across the health wellness-illness continuum to at least one population focus as defined by nationally recognized role and population-focused competencies; however, the emphasis and implementation within each APRN role varies. The services or care provided by APRNs is not defined or limited by setting but rather by patient care needs. The continuum encompasses the range of health states from homeostasis (or wellness) to a disruption in the state of health in which basic needs are not met or maintained (illness), with health problems of varying acuity occurring along the continuum that must be prevented or resolved to maintain wellness or an optimal level of functioning (WHO, 2006). Although all APRNs are educationally prepared to provide care to patients across the health wellness-illness continuum, the emphasis and how implemented within each APRN role varies.

The Certified Registered Nurse Anesthetist
The Certified Registered Nurse Anesthetist is prepared to provide the full spectrum of patients' anesthesia care and anesthesia-related care for individuals across the lifespan, whose health status may range from healthy through all recognized levels of acuity, including persons with immediate, severe, or life-threatening illnesses or injury. This care is provided in diverse settings, including hospital surgical suites and obstetrical delivery rooms; critical access hospitals; acute care; pain management centers; ambulatory surgical centers; and the offices of dentists, podiatrists, ophthalmologists, and plastic surgeons.

The Certified Nurse-Midwife
The certified nurse-midwife provides a full range of primary health care services to women throughout the lifespan, including gynecologic care, family planning services, preconception care, prenatal and postpartum care, childbirth, and care of the newborn. The practice includes treating the male partner of their female clients for sexually transmitted disease and reproductive health. This care is provided in diverse settings, which may include home, hospital, birth center, and a variety of ambulatory care settings including private offices and community and public health clinics.

The Clinical Nurse Specialist
The CNS has a unique APRN role to integrate care across the continuum and through three spheres of influence: patient, nurse, system. The three spheres are overlapping and interrelated but each sphere possesses a distinctive focus. In each of the spheres of influence, the primary goal of the CNS is continuous improvement of patient outcomes and nursing care. Key elements of CNS practice are to create environments through mentoring and

8

APRN Joint Dialogue Group Report, July 7, 2008

system changes that empower nurses to develop caring, evidence-based practices to alleviate patient distress, facilitate ethical decision-making, and respond to diversity. The CNS is responsible and accountable for diagnosis and treatment of health/illness states, disease management, health promotion, and prevention of illness and risk behaviors among individuals, families, groups, and communities.

The Certified Nurse Practitioner

For the certified nurse practitioner (CNP), care along the wellness-illness continuum is a dynamic process in which direct primary and acute care is provided across settings. CNPs are members of the health delivery system, practicing autonomously in areas as diverse as family practice, pediatrics, internal medicine, geriatrics, and women's health care. CNPs are prepared to diagnose and treat patients with undifferentiated symptoms as well as those with established diagnoses. Both primary and acute care CNPs provide initial, ongoing, and comprehensive care, includes taking comprehensive histories, providing physical examinations and other health assessment and screening activities, and diagnosing, treating, and managing patients with acute and chronic illnesses and diseases. This includes ordering, performing, supervising, and interpreting laboratory and imaging studies; prescribing medication and durable medical equipment; and making appropriate referrals for patients and families. Clinical CNP care includes health promotion, disease prevention, health education, and counseling as well as the diagnosis and management of acute and chronic diseases. Certified nurse practitioners are prepared to practice as primary care CNPs and acute care CNPs, which have separate national consensus-based competencies and separate certification processes.

Titling

The title Advanced Practice Registered Nurse (APRN) is the licensing title to be used for the subset of nurses prepared with advanced, graduate-level nursing knowledge to provide direct patient care in four roles: certified registered nurse anesthetist, certified nurse-midwife, clinical nurse specialist, and certified nurse practitioner.[4] This title, APRN, is a legally protected title. Licensure and scope of practice are based on graduate education in one of the four roles and in a defined population.

Verification of licensure, whether hard copy or electronic, will indicate the role and population for which the APRN has been licensed.

At a minimum, an individual must legally represent themselves, including in a legal signature, as an APRN and by the role. He/she may indicate the population as well. No one, except those who are licensed to practice as an APRN, may use the APRN title or any of the APRN role titles. An individual also may add the specialty title in which they are professionally recognized in addition to the legal title of APRN and role.

---

[4] Nurses with advanced graduate nursing preparation practicing in roles and specialties that do not provide direct care to individuals and, therefore, whose practice does not require regulatory recognition beyond the Registered Nurse license granted by state boards of nursing may not use any term or title which may confuse the public, including advanced practice nurse or advanced practice registered nurse. The term *advanced public health nursing* however, may be used to identify nurses practicing in this advanced specialty area of nursing.

9

APRN Joint Dialogue Group Report, July 7, 2008

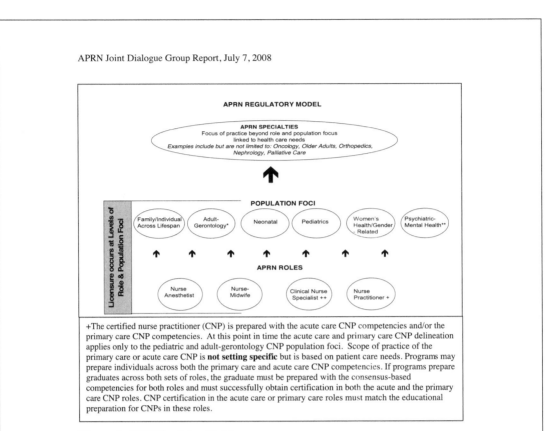

+The certified nurse practitioner (CNP) is prepared with the acute care CNP competencies and/or the primary care CNP competencies. At this point in time the acute care and primary care CNP delineation applies only to the pediatric and adult-gerontology CNP population foci. Scope of practice of the primary care or acute care CNP is **not setting specific** but is based on patient care needs. Programs may prepare individuals across both the primary care and acute care CNP competencies. If programs prepare graduates across both sets of roles, the graduate must be prepared with the consensus-based competencies for both roles and must successfully obtain certification in both the acute and the primary care CNP roles. CNP certification in the acute care or primary care roles must match the educational preparation for CNPs in these roles.

Diagram 1: APRN Regulatory Model

Under this APRN Regulatory Model, there are four roles: certified registered nurse anesthetist (CRNA), certified nurse-midwife (CNM), clinical nurse specialist (CNS), and certified nurse practitioner (CNP). These four roles are given the title of advanced practice registered nurse (APRN). APRNs are educated in one of the four roles and in at least one of six population foci: family/individual across the lifespan, adult-gerontology, neonatal, pediatrics, women's health/gender-related or psych/mental health. Individuals will be licensed as independent practitioners for practice at the level of one of the four APRN roles within at least one of the six identified population foci. Education, certification, and licensure of an individual must be congruent in terms of role and population foci. APRNs may specialize but they can not be licensed solely within a specialty area. Specialties can provide depth in one's practice within the established population foci.

* The population focus, adult-gerontology, encompasses the young adult to the older adult, including the frail elderly. APRNs educated and certified in the adult-gerontology population are educated and certified across both areas of practice and will be titled Adult-Gerontology CNP or CNS. In addition, all APRNs in any of the four roles providing care to the adult population, e.g., family or gender specific, must be prepared to meet the growing needs of the older adult population. Therefore, the education program should include didactic and clinical education experiences necessary to prepare APRNs with these enhanced skills and knowledge.
** The population focus, psychiatric/mental health, encompasses education and practice across the lifespan.
++ The Clinical Nurse Specialist (CNS) is educated and assessed through national certification processes across the continuum from wellness through acute care.

10

APRN Joint Dialogue Group Report, July 7, 2008

Broad-based APRN Education

For entry into APRN practice and for regulatory purposes, APRN education must:

- be formal education with a graduate degree or post-graduate certificate (either post-master's or post-doctoral) that is awarded by an academic institution and accredited by a nursing or nursing-related accrediting organization recognized by the U.S. Department of Education (USDE) and/or the Council for Higher Education Accreditation (CHEA);
- be awarded pre-approval, pre-accreditation, or accreditation status prior to admitting students;
- be comprehensive and at the graduate level;
- prepare the graduate to practice in one of the four identified APRN roles;
- prepare the graduate with the core competencies for one of the APRN roles across *at least one* of the six population foci;
- include at a minimum, three separate comprehensive *graduate-level* courses (the APRN Core) in:
  - o Advanced physiology/pathophysiology, including general principles that apply across the lifespan;
  - o Advanced health assessment, which includes assessment of all human systems, advanced assessment techniques, concepts and approaches; and
  - o Advanced pharmacology, which includes pharmacodynamics, pharmacokinetics and pharmacotherapeutics of all broad categories of agents.
- Additional content, specific to the role and population, in these three APRN core areas should be integrated throughout the other role and population didactic and clinical courses;
- Provide a basic understanding of the principles for decision making in the identified role;
- Prepare the graduate to assume responsibility and accountability for health promotion and/or maintenance as well as the assessment, diagnosis, and management of patient problems, which includes the use and prescription of pharmacologic and non-pharmacologic interventions; and
- Ensure clinical and didactic coursework is comprehensive and sufficient to prepare the graduate to practice in the APRN role and population focus.

Preparation in a specialty area of practice is optional but if included must build on the APRN role/population-focus competencies. Clinical and didactic coursework must be comprehensive and sufficient to prepare the graduate to obtain certification for licensure in and to practice in the APRN role and population focus.

As part of the accreditation process, all APRN education programs must undergo a pre-approval, pre-accreditation, or accreditation process prior to admitting students. The purpose of the pre-approval process is twofold: 1) to ensure that students graduating from the program will be able to meet the education criteria necessary for national certification in the role and population-focus and if successfully certified, are eligible for licensure to practice in the APRN role/population-focus; and 2) to ensure that programs will meet all educational standards prior to starting the program. The pre-approval, pre-accreditation or accreditation processes may vary across APRN roles.

11

APRN Joint Dialogue Group Report, July 7, 2008

APRN Specialties

Preparation in a specialty area of practice is optional, but if included must build on the APRN role/population-focused competencies. Specialty practice represents a much more focused area of preparation and practice than does the APRN role/population focus level. Specialty practice may focus on specific patient populations beyond those identified or health care needs such as oncology, palliative care, substance abuse, or nephrology. The criteria for defining an APRN specialty is built upon the ANA (2004) Criteria for Recognition as a Nursing Specialty (see Appendix B). APRN specialty education and practice build upon and are in addition to the education and practice of the APRN role and population focus. For example, a family CNP could specialize in elder care or nephrology; an Adult-Gerontology CNS could specialize in palliative care; a CRNA could specialize in pain management; or a CNM could specialize in care of the post-menopausal woman. State licensing boards will not regulate the APRN at the level of specialties in this APRN Regulatory Model. Professional certification in the specialty area of practice is strongly recommended.

An APRN specialty
* preparation cannot replace educational preparation in the role or one of the six population foci;
* preparation can not expand one's scope of practice beyond the role or population focus
* addresses a subset of the population-focus;
* title may not be used in lieu of the licensing title, which includes the role or role/population; and
* is developed, recognized, and monitored by the profession.

New specialties emerge based on health needs of the population. APRN specialties develop to provide added value to the role practice as well as providing flexibility within the profession to meet these emerging needs of patients. Specialties also may cross several or all APRN roles. A specialty evolves out of an APRN role/population focus and indicates that an APRN has *additional* knowledge and expertise in a more discrete area of specialty practice. Competency in the specialty areas could be acquired either by educational preparation or experience and assessed in a variety of ways through professional credentialing mechanisms (e.g., portfolios, examinations, etc.).

Education programs may concurrently prepare individuals in a specialty providing they meet all of the other requirements for APRN education programs, including preparation in the APRN core, role, and population core competencies. In addition, for licensure purposes, one exam must assess the APRN core, role, and population-focused competencies. For example, a nurse anesthetist would write one certification examination, which tests the APRN core, CRNA role, and population-focused competencies, administered by the Council on Certification for Nurse Anesthetist; or a primary care family nurse practitioner would write one certification examination, which tests the APRN core, CNP role, and family population-focused competencies, administered by ANCC or AANP. Specialty competencies must be assessed separately. In summary, education programs preparing individuals with this additional knowledge in a specialty, *if used for entry into advanced practice registered nursing and for regulatory purposes*, must also prepare individuals in one of the four nationally recognized APRN roles and in one of the six population foci. Individuals must be

12

APRN Joint Dialogue Group Report, July 7, 2008

recognized and credentialed in one of the four APRN roles within at least one population foci. APRNs are licensed at the role/population focus level and **not** at the specialty level. However, if not intended for entry-level preparation in one of the four roles/population foci and not for regulatory purposes, education programs, using a variety of formats and methodologies, may provide licensed APRNs with the additional knowledge, skills, and abilities, to become professionally certified in the specialty area of APRN practice.

Emergence of New APRN Roles and Population-Foci

As nursing practice evolves and health care needs of the population change, new APRN roles or population-foci may evolve over time. An APRN role would encompass a unique or significantly differentiated set of competencies from any of the other APRN roles. In addition, the scope of practice within the role or population focus is not entirely subsumed within one of the other roles. Careful consideration of new APRN roles or population-foci is in the best interest of the profession.

For licensure, there must be clear guidance for national recognition of a new APRN role or population-focus. A new role or population focus should be discussed and vetted through the national licensure, accreditation, certification, education communication structure: LACE. An essential part of being recognized as a role or population-focus is that educational standards and practice competencies must exist, be consistent, and must be nationally recognized by the profession. Characteristics of the process to be used to develop nationally recognized core competencies, and education and practice standards for a newly emerging role or population-focus are:

1. national in scope
2. inclusive
3. transparent
4. accountable
5. initiated by nursing
6. consistent with national standards for licensure, accreditation, certification and education
7. evidence-based
8. consistent with regulatory principles.

To be recognized, an APRN role must meet the following criteria:

- nationally recognized education standards and core competencies for programs preparing individuals in the role;
- education programs, including graduate degree granting (master's, doctoral) and post-graduate certificate programs, are accredited by a nursing or nursing-related accrediting organization that is recognized by the U.S. Department of Education (USDE) and/or the Council for Higher Education Accreditation (CHEA); and
- professional nursing certification program that is psychometrically sound, legally defensible, and which meets nationally recognized accreditation standards for certification programs.[5]

---

[5] The professional certification program should be nationally accredited by the American Board of Nursing Specialties (ABNS) or the National Commission for Certifying Agencies (NCCA).

13

APRN Joint Dialogue Group Report, July 7, 2008

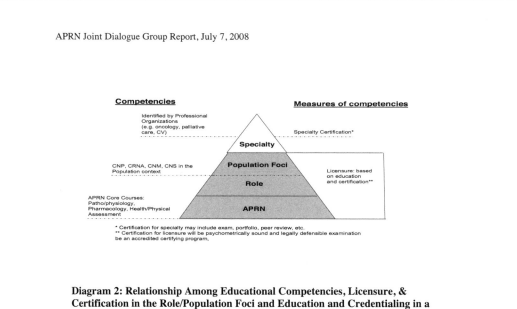

Diagram 2: Relationship Among Educational Competencies, Licensure, & Certification in the Role/Population Foci and Education and Credentialing in a Specialty

IMPLEMENTATION STRATEGIES FOR APRN REGULATORY MODEL

In order to accomplish the above model, the four prongs of regulation: licensure, accreditation, certification, and education (LACE) must work together. Expectations for licensure, accreditation, certification, and education are listed below:

Foundational Requirements for Licensure
Boards of nursing will:
1. license APRNs in the categories of Certified Registered Nurse Anesthetist, Certified Nurse-Midwife, Clinical Nurse Specialist or Certified Nurse Practitioner within a specific population focus;
2. be solely responsible for licensing Advanced Practice Registered Nurses[6];
3. only license graduates of accredited graduate programs that prepare graduates with the APRN core, role and population competencies;
4. require successful completion of a national certification examination that assesses APRN core, role and population competencies for APRN licensure.
5. not issue a temporary license;
6. only license an APRN when education and certification are congruent;
7. license APRNs as independent practitioners with no regulatory requirements for collaboration, direction or supervision;
8. allow for mutual recognition of advanced practice registered nursing through the APRN Compact;

---

[6] Except in states where state boards of nurse-midwifery or midwifery regulate nurse-midwives or nurse-midwives and midwives jointly.

14

APRN Joint Dialogue Group Report, July 7, 2008

9. have at least one APRN representative position on the board and utilize an APRN advisory committee that includes representatives of all four APRN roles; and,

10. institute a grandfathering[7] clause that will exempt those APRNs already practicing in the state from new eligibility requirements.

Foundational Requirements for Accreditation of Education Programs

Accreditors will:

1. be responsible for evaluating APRN education programs including graduate degree-granting and post-graduate certificate programs.[8].

2. through their established accreditation standards and process, assess APRN education programs in light of the APRN core, role core, and population core competencies;

3. assess developing APRN education programs and tracks by reviewing them using established accreditation standards and granting pre-approval, pre-accreditation, or accreditation prior to student enrollment;

4. include an APRN on the visiting team when an APRN program/track is being reviewed; and

5. monitor APRN educational programs throughout the accreditation period by reviewing them using established accreditation standards and processes.

Foundational Requirements for Certification

Certification programs providing APRN certification used for licensure will:

1. follow established certification testing and psychometrically sound, legally defensible standards for APRN examinations for licensure (see appendix A for the NCSBN Criteria for APRN Certification Programs);

2. assess the APRN core and role competencies across at least one population focus of practice;

3. assess specialty competencies, if appropriate, separately from the APRN core, role and population-focused competencies;

4. be accredited by a national certification accreditation body;[9]

---

[7] Grandfathering is a provision in a new law exempting those already in or a part of the existing system that is being regulated. When states adopt new eligibility requirements for APRNs, currently practicing APRNs will be permitted to continue practicing within the state(s) of their current licensure.
However, if an APRN applies for licensure by endorsement in another state, the APRN would be eligible for licensure if s/he demonstrates that the following criteria have been met:
- current, active practice in the advanced role and population focus area,
- current active, national certification or recertification, as applicable, in the advanced role and population focus area,
- compliance with the APRN educational requirements of the state in which the APRN is applying for licensure that were in effect at the time the APRN completed his/her APRN education program, and
- compliance with all other criteria set forth by the state in which the APRN is applying for licensure (e.g. recent CE, RN licensure).
Once the model has been adopted and implemented (date to be determined by the state boards of nursing. See proposed timeline on page 14-15.) all new graduates applying for APRN licensure must meet the requirements outlined in this regulatory model
[8] Degree-granting programs include both master's and doctoral programs. Post-graduate certificate programs include post-master's and post-doctoral education programs.
[9] The certification program should be nationally accredited by the American Board of Nursing Specialties (ABNS) or the National Commission for Certifying Agencies (NCCA).

15

APRN Joint Dialogue Group Report, July 7, 2008

5. enforce congruence (role and population focus) between the education program and the type of certification examination;
6. provide a mechanism to ensure ongoing competence and maintenance of certification;
7. participate in ongoing relationships which make their processes transparent to boards of nursing;
8. participate in a mutually agreeable mechanism to ensure communication with boards of nursing and schools of nursing.

Foundational Requirements for Education

APRN education programs/tracks leading to APRN licensure, including graduate degree-granting and post-graduate certificate programs will:
1. follow established educational standards and ensure attainment of the APRN core, role core and population core competencies [10,11]
2. be accredited by a nursing accrediting organization that is recognized by the U.S. Department of Education (USDE) and/or the Council for Higher Education Accreditation (CHEA). [12]
3. be pre-approved, pre-accredited, or accredited prior to the acceptance of students, including all developing APRN education programs and tracks;
4. ensure that graduates of the program are eligible for national certification and state licensure; and
5. ensure that official documentation (e.g., transcript) specifies the role and population focus of the graduate.

Communication Strategies

A formal communication mechanism, LACE, which includes those regulatory organizations that represent APRN licensure, accreditation, certification, and education entities would be created. The purpose of LACE would be to provide a formal, ongoing communication mechanism that provides for transparent and aligned communication among the identified entities. The collaborative efforts between the APRN Consensus Group and the NCSBN APRN Advisory Panel, through the APRN Joint Dialogue Group have illustrated the ongoing level of communication necessary among these groups to ensure that all APRN stakeholders are involved. Several strategies including equal representation on an integrated board with

---

[10] The APRN core competencies for all APRN nursing education programs located in schools of nursing are delineated in the American Association of Colleges of Nursing (1996) *The Essentials of Master's Education for Advanced Practice Nursing Education* or the AACN (2006) *The Essentials of Doctoral Education for Advanced Nursing Practice*. The APRN core competencies for nurse anesthesia and nurse-midwifery education programs located outside of a school of nursing are delineated by the accrediting organizations for their respective roles i.e., Council on Accreditation of Nurse Anesthesia Educational Programs (COA), Accreditation Commission for Midwifery Education (ACME).
[11] APRN programs outside of schools of nursing must prepare graduates with the APRN core which includes three separate graduate-level courses in pathophysiology/physiology, health assessment, and pharmacology.
[12] APRN education programs must be accredited by a nursing accrediting organization that is recognized by the U.S. Department of Education (USDE) and/or the Council for Higher Education Accreditation (CHEA), including the Commission on Collegiate Nursing Education (CCNE), National League for Nursing Accrediting Commission (NLNAC), Council on Accreditation of Nurse Anesthesia Educational Programs (COA), Accreditation Commission for Midwifery Education (ACME), and the National Association of Nurse Practitioners in Women's Health Council on Accreditation.

16

APRN Joint Dialogue Group Report, July 7, 2008

face-to-face meetings, audio and teleconferencing, pass-protected access to agency web sites, and regular reporting mechanisms have been recommended. These strategies will build trust and enhance information sharing. Examples of issues to be addressed by the group would be: guaranteeing appropriate representation of APRN roles among accreditation site visitors, documentation of program completion by education institutions, notification of examination outcomes to educators and regulators, notification of disciplinary action toward licensees by boards of nursing.

Creating the LACE Structure and Processes

Several principles should guide the formulation of a structure including: 1) all four entities of LACE should have representation; 2) the total should allow effective discussion of and response to issues and ; 3) the structure should not be duplicative of existing structures such as the Alliance for APRN Credentialing. Consideration should be given to evolving the existing Alliance structure to meet the needs of LACE. Guidance from an organizational consultant will be useful in forming a permanent structure that will endure and support the work that needs to continue. The new structure will support fair decision-making among all relevant stakeholders. In addition, the new structure will be in place as soon as possible.

The LACE organizational structure should include representation of:
- State licensing boards, including at least one compact and one non-compact state;
- Accrediting bodies that accredit education programs of the four APRN roles;
- Certifying bodies that offer APRN certification used for regulatory purposes; and,
- Education organizations that set standards for APRN education.

Timeline for Implementation of Regulatory Model

Implementation of the recommendations for an APRN Regulatory Model will occur incrementally. Due to the interdependence of licensure, accreditation, certification, and education, certain recommendations will be implemented sequentially. However, recognizing that this model was developed through a consensus process with participation of APRN certifiers, accreditors, public regulators, educators, and employers, it is expected that the recommendations and model delineated will inform decisions made by each of these entities as the APRN community moves to fully implement the APRN Regulatory Model. A target date for full implementation of the Regulatory Model and all embedded recommendations is the Year 2015.

HISTORICAL BACKGROUND

NCSBN APRN Committee (previously APRN Advisory Panel)

NCSBN became involved with advanced practice nursing when boards of nursing began using the results of APRN certification examinations as one of the requirements for APRN licensure. During the 1993 NCSBN annual meeting, delegates adopted a position paper on the licensure of advanced nursing practice which included model legislation language and model administrative rules for advanced nursing practice. NCSBN core competencies for certified nurse practitioners were adopted the following year.

17

APRN Joint Dialogue Group Report, July 7, 2008

In 1995, NCSBN was directed by the Delegate Assembly to work with APRN certifiers to make certification examinations suitable for regulatory purposes. Since then, much effort has been made toward that purpose. During the mid and late 90's, the APRN certifiers agreed to undergo accreditation and provide additional information to boards of nursing to ensure that their examinations were psychometrically sound and legally defensible (NCSBN, 1998).

During the early 2000s, the APRN Advisory Panel developed criteria for ARPN certification programs and for accreditations agencies. In January 2002, the board of directors approved the criteria and process for a new review process for APRN certification programs. The criteria represented required elements of certification programs that would result in a legally defensible examination suitable for the regulation of advanced practice nurses. Subsequently, the APRN Advisory Panel has worked with certification programs to improve the legal defensibility of APRN certification examinations and to promote communication with all APRN stakeholders regarding APRN regulatory issues such as with the establishment of the annual NCSBN APRN Roundtable in the mid 1990's. In 2002, the Advisory Panel also developed a position paper describing APRN regulatory issues of concern.

In 2003, the APRN Advisory Panel began a draft APRN vision paper in an attempt to resolve APRN regulatory concerns such as the proliferation of APRN subspecialty areas. The purpose of the APRN Vision Paper was to provide direction to boards of nursing regarding APRN regulation for the next 8-10 years by identifying an ideal future APRN regulatory model. Eight recommendations were made. The draft vision paper was completed in 2006. After reviewing the draft APRN vision paper at their February 2006 board meeting, the board of directors directed that the paper be disseminated to boards of nursing and APRN stakeholders for feedback. The Vision paper also was discussed during the 2006 APRN Roundtable. The large response from boards of nursing and APRN stakeholders was varied. The APRN Advisory Panel spent the remaining part of 2006, reviewing and discussing the feedback with APRN stakeholders. (See Appendix C for the list of APRN Advisory Panel members who worked on the draft APRN Vision Paper and Appendix D for the list of organizations represented at the 2006 APRN Roundtable where the draft vision paper was presented.)

APRN Consensus Group

In March 2004, the American Association of Colleges of Nursing (AACN) and the National Organization of Nurse Practitioner Faculties (NONPF) submitted a proposal to the Alliance for Nursing Accreditation, now named Alliance for APRN Credentialing[13] (hereafter referred to as *the APRN Alliance*) to establish a process to develop a consensus[14] statement on the credentialing of advanced practice nurses (APNs).[15] The APRN Alliance[16], created in 1997,

---

[13] At its March 2006 meeting, the Alliance for Nursing Accreditation voted to change its name to the Alliance for APRN Credentialing which more accurately reflects its membership.
[14] The goal of the APRN Work Group was unanimous agreement on all issues and recommendations. However, this was recognized as an unrealistic expectation and may delay the process; therefore, consensus was defined as a two thirds majority agreement by those members of the Work Group present at the table as organizational representatives with each participating organization having one vote.
[15] The term advanced practice nurse (APN) was initially used by the Work Group and is used in this section of the report to accurately reflect the background discussion. However, the Work group reached consensus that the term advanced practice registered nurse (APRN) should be adopted for use in subsequent discussions and documents.

18

APRN Joint Dialogue Group Report, July 7, 2008

was convened by AACN to regularly discuss issues related to nursing education, practice, and credentialing. A number of differing views on how APN practice is defined, what constitutes specialization versus subspecialization, and the appropriate credentialing requirements that would authorize practice had emerged over the past several years.

An invitation to participate in a national APN consensus process was sent to 50 organizations that were identified as having an interest in advanced practice nursing (see Appendix F). Thirty-two organizations participated in the APN Consensus Conference in Washington, D.C. June 2004. The focus of the one-day meeting was to initiate an in-depth examination of issues related to APN definition, specialization, sub-specialization, and regulation, which includes accreditation, education, certification, and licensure[17]. Based on recommendations generated in the June 2004 APN Consensus Conference, the Alliance formed a smaller work group made up of designees from 23 organizations with broad representation of APN certification, licensure, education, accreditation, and practice. The charge to the work group was to develop a statement that addresses the issues, delineated during the APN Consensus Conference with the goal of envisioning a future model for APNs. The Alliance APN Consensus Work Group (hereafter referred to as *the Work Group*) convened for 16 days of intensive discussion between October 2004 and July 2007 (see Appendix H for a list of organizations represented on the APN Work Group).

In December 2004, the American Nurses Association (ANA) and AACN co-hosted an APN stakeholder meeting to address those issues identified at the June 2004 APN Consensus meeting. Attendees agreed to ask the APN Work Group to continue to craft a consensus statement that would include recommendations regarding APN regulation, specialization, and subspecialization. It also was agreed that organizations in attendance who had not participated in the June 2004 APN Consensus meeting would be included in the APN Consensus Group and that this larger group would reconvene at a future date to discuss the recommendations of the APN Work Group.

Following the December 2004 APN Consensus meeting, the Work Group continued to work diligently to reach consensus on the issues surrounding APRN education, practice, accreditation, certification, and licensure, and to create a future consensus-based model for APRN regulation. Subsequent APRN Consensus Group meetings were held in September 2005 and June 2006. All organizations who participated in the APRN Consensus Group are listed in Appendix G.

---

[16] Organizational members of the Alliance for APRN Credentialing : American Academy of Nurse Practitioners Certification Program, American Association of Colleges of Nursing, American Association of Critical-Care Nurses Certification Corporation, Council on Accreditation of Nurse Anesthesia Educational Programs, American College of Nurse-Midwives, American Nurses Credentialing Center, Association of Faculties of Pediatric Nurse Practitioners, Inc., Commission on Collegiate Nursing Education, National Association of Clinical Nurse Specialists, National Association of Nurse Practitioners in Women's Health, Council on Accreditation, Pediatric Nursing Certification Board, The National Certification Corporation for the Obstetric Gynecologic and Neonatal Nursing Specialties, National Council of State Boards of Nursing, National Organization of Nurse Practitioner Faculties

[17] The term regulation refers to the four prongs of regulation: licensure, accreditation, certification and education.

19

APRN Joint Dialogue Group Report, July 7, 2008

APRN Joint Dialogue Group

In April, 2006, the APRN Advisory Panel met with the APRN Consensus Work Group to discuss APRN issues described in the NCSBN draft vision paper. The APRN Consensus Work Group requested and was provided with feedback from the APRN Advisory Panel regarding the APRN Consensus Group Report. Both groups agreed to continue to dialogue.

As the APRN Advisory Panel and APRN Consensus Work Group continued their work in parallel fashion, concerns regarding the need for each group's work not to conflict with the other were expressed. A subgroup of seven people from the APRN Consensus Work Group and seven individuals from the APRN Advisory Panel were convened in January, 2007. The group called itself the APRN Joint Dialogue Group (see Appendix E) and the agenda consisted of discussing areas of agreement and disagreement between the two groups. The goal of the subgroup meetings was anticipated to be two papers that did not conflict, but rather complemented each other. However, as the APRN Joint Dialogue Group continued to meet, much progress was made regarding areas of agreement; it was determined that rather than two papers being disseminated, one joint paper would be developed, which reflected the work of both groups. This document is the product of the work of the APRN Joint Dialogue Group and through the consensus-based work of the APRN Consensus Work Group and the NCSBN APRN Advisory Committee.

Assumptions Underlying the Work of the Joint Dialogue Group

The consensus-based recommendations that have emerged from the extensive dialogue and consensus-based processes delineated in this report are based on the following assumptions:

- Recommendations must address current issues facing the advanced practice registered nurse (APRN) community but should be future oriented.
- The ultimate goal of licensure, accreditation, certification, and education is to promote patient safety and public protection.
- The recognition that this document was developed with the participation of APRN certifiers, accreditors, public regulators, educators, and employers. The intention is that the document will allow for informed decisions made by each of these entities as they address APRN issues.

CONCLUSION

The recommendations offered in this paper present an APRN regulatory model as a collaborative effort among APRN educators, accreditors, certifiers, and licensure bodies. The essential elements of APRN regulation are identified as licensure, accreditation, certification, and education. The recommendations reflect a need and desire to collaborate among regulatory bodies to achieve a sound model and continued communication with the goal of increasing the clarity and uniformity of APRN regulation.

The goals of the consensus processes were to:

- strive for harmony and common understanding in the APRN regulatory community that would continue to promote quality APRN education and practice;
- develop a vision for APRN regulation, including education, accreditation, certification, and licensure;

20

APRN Joint Dialogue Group Report, July 7, 2008

- establish a set of standards that protect the public, improve mobility, and improve access to safe, quality APRN care; and
- produce a written statement that reflects consensus on APRN regulatory issues.

In summary, this report includes: a definition of the APRN Regulatory Model, including a definition of the Advanced Practice Registered Nurse; a definition of broad-based APRN education; a model for regulation that ensures APRN education and certification as a valid and reliable process, that is based on nationally recognized and accepted standards; uniform recommendations for licensing bodies across states; a process and characteristics for recognizing a new APRN role; and a definition of an APRN specialty that allows for the profession to meet future patient and nursing needs.

The work of the Joint Dialogue Group in conjunction with all organizations representing APRN licensure, accreditation, certification, and education to advance a regulatory model is an ongoing collaborative process that is fluid and dynamic. As health care evolves and new standards and needs emerge, the APRN Regulatory Model will advance accordingly to allow APRNs to care for patients in a safe environment to the full potential of their nursing knowledge and skill.

21

APRN Joint Dialogue Group Report, July 7, 2008

REFERENCES

American Association of Colleges of Nursing. (1996). *The Essentials of Master's Education for Advanced Practice Nursing Education*. Washington, DC: Author

.
American Association of Colleges of Nursing. (2004). *Position Statement on the Practice Doctorate in Nursing*. Washington, DC: Author. Accessed at http://www.aacn.nche.edu/DNP/DNPPositionStatement.htm.

American Association of Colleges of Nursing. (2006). *The Essentials of Doctoral Education for Advanced Nursing Practice*. Washington, DC: Author.

American College of Nurse-Midwives (2002). Core Competencies for Basic Midwifery Practice. Accessed at http://www.midwife.org/display.cfm?id=137.

American Educational Research Association, American Psychological Association and National Council on Measurement in Education (2002). "Professional and Occupational Licensure and Certification: Standards for Educational and Psychological Testing, Washington, D.C.: American Psychological Association, Inc.

American Nurses Association. (2004). *Nursing: Scope and Standards of Practice*. Washington, DC: Author.

Association of Women's Health, Obstetric and Neonatal Nurses & National Association of Nurse Practitioners Women's Health (2002). *The Women's Health Nurse Practitioner: Guidelines for Practice and Education, 5th edition*. Washington, DC: Author

Atkinson, Dale J. (2000). Legal issues in Licensure Policy. In Schoon, Craig, & Smith I. Lion (eds.) *The Licensure and Certification Mission: Legal, Social, and Political Foundations. Professional Examination Service*. New York.

Barbara J. Safriet on "Health Care Dollars & Regulatory Sense: The Role of Advanced Practice Nursing", *Yale Journal on Regulation*, Vol., No. 2, 447.

Bauer, Jeffrey. (1998). *Not What the Doctor Ordered: How to End the Medical Monopoly in the Pursuit of Managed Care 2nd ed*. McGraw-Hill Companies: New York.

Citizen Advocacy Center (2004). *Maintaining and Improving Health Professional Competence; Roadway to Continuing Competency Assurance*.

Council on Accreditation of Nurse Anesthesia Educational Programs. (2004). *Standards for Accreditation of Nurse Anesthesia Educational Programs*. Chicago: Author.

Finocchio, L.J., Dower, C.M., Blick N.T., Gragnola, C.M., & The Taskforce on Health Care Workforce Regulation. (1998). *Strengthening Consumer Protection: Priorities for Health Care Workforce Regulation*. San Francisco, CA: Pew Health Professions Commission.

22

APRN Joint Dialogue Group Report, July 7, 2008

Hamric, Ann B. & Hanson, Charlene (2003). Educating Advanced Practice Nurses for Practice Reality. *Journal of Professional Nursing, 19,* No 5 (September-October) 262-268.

Hanson, C. & Hamric, Ann. (2003). Reflections on the continuing Evolution of Advanced Practice Nursing. *Nursing Outlook. 51.* No. 5 (September/October) 203-211.

Institute of Medicine (2003). *Health Professions Education: A Bridge to Quality.* Board on Health Care Services.

Kaplan, Louise, & Brown, Marie-Annette (2004). Prescriptive Authority and Barriers to NP Practice. *The Nurse Practitioner, 29,* No. 33, 28-35.

Marion, Lucy, et all (2003). The Practice Doctorate in Nursing: Future or Fringe. *Topics in Advanced Practice Nursing eJournal 3*(2).2003 @ 2003 Medscape.

National Association of Clinical Nurse Specialists (2003). *Statement on Clinical Nurse Specialist Practice.*

National Council of State Boards of Nursing (1993). *Regulation of Advanced Practice Nursing: 1993 National Council of State Boards of Nursing Position Paper.* Chicago: Author

National Council of State Boards of Nursing (1997). *The National Council of State Boards of Nursing Position Paper on Approval and Accreditation: Definition and Usage.* Chicago: Author

National Council of State Boards of Nursing (1998). *Using Nurse Practitioner Certification for State Nursing Regulation: A Historical Perspective.* Chicago: Author

National Council of State Boards of Nursing (2001). *Advanced Practice Registered Nurse Compact.* Chicago: Author

National Council of State Boards of Nursing (2002). *Regulation of Advanced Practice Nursing: 2002 National Council of State Boards of Nursing Position Paper.* Chicago: Author.

National Council of State Boards of Nursing (2002). *Uniform Advanced Practice Registered Nurse Licensure/Authority to Practice Requirements.* Chicago: Author.

National Council of State Boards of Nursing. (2002). *Regulation of Advanced Practice Nursing.* Printed from http://www.ncsbn.org. Chicago, IL: Author.

National Organization of Nurse Practitioner Faculties. (2000). *Domains and Competencies of Nurse Practitioner Practice.* Washington, DC: Author.

National Panel for Acute Care Nurse Practitioner Competencies. (2004). *Acute Care Nurse Practitioner Competencies.* Washington, DC: NONPF

23

APRN Joint Dialogue Group Report, July 7, 2008

National Panel for Psychiatric-Mental Health NP Competencies. (2003). *Psychiatric-Mental Health Nurse Practitioner Competencies*. Washington, DC: NONPF

National Task Force on Quality Nurse Practitioner Education. (2002). *Criteria for Evaluation of Nurse Practitioner Programs*. Washington, DC: NONPF

Pew Health Professions Commission (1995). *Critical Challenges: Revitalizing The Health Professions for the Twenty-First Century*. National Academies Press, Washington, D.C.

World Health Organization. (2006). *WHO Health Promotion Glossary: new terms*. *Health Promotion International Advance Access*. Oxford University Press: Author. Can be accessed at http://www.who.int/healthpromotion/about/HP%20Glossay%20in%20HPI.pdf.

24

APRN Joint Dialogue Group Report, July 7, 2008

APPENDIX A
NCSBN CRITERIA FOR EVALUATING CERTIFICATION PROGRAMS

Criteria	Elaboration
I. The program is national in the scope of its credentialing.	A. The advanced nursing practice category and standards of practice have been identified by national organizations. B. Credentialing services are available to nurses throughout the United States and its territories. C. There is a provision for public representation on the certification board. D. A nursing specialty organization that establishes standards for the nursing specialty exists. E. A tested body of knowledge related to the advanced practice nursing specialty exists. F. The certification board is an entity with organizational autonomy.

II. Conditions for taking the examination are consistent with acceptable standards of the testing community.	A. Applicants do not have to belong to an affiliated professional organization in order to apply for certification offered by the certification program.
	B. Eligibility criteria rationally related to competence to practice safely.
	C. Published criteria are enforced.
	D. In compliance with the American Disabilities Act.
	E. Sample application(s) are available.
	   1) Certification requirements included
	   2) Application procedures include:
	      • procedures for ensuring match between education and clinical experience, and APRN specialty being certified,
	      • procedures for validating information provided by candidate,
	      • procedures for handling omissions and discrepancies
	   3) Professional staff responsible for credential review and admission decisions.
	   4) Examination should be administered frequently enough to be accessible but not so frequently as to over-expose items.
	F. Periodic review of eligibility criteria and application procedures to ensure that they are fair and equitable.

III. Educational requirements are consistent with the requirements of the advanced practice specialty.	A. Current U.S. registered nurse licensure is required.
	B. Graduation from a graduate advanced practice education program meets the following requirements:
	   1) Education program offered by an accredited college or university offers a graduate degree with a concentration in the advanced nursing practice specialty the individual is seeking
	   2) If post-masters certificate programs are offered, they must be offered through institutions meeting criteria B.1.
	   3) Both direct and indirect clinical supervision must be congruent with current national specialty organizations and nursing

25

APRN Joint Dialogue Group Report, July 7, 2008

	accreditation guidelines
	4) The curriculum includes, but is not limited to:
	• biological, behavioral, medical, and nursing sciences relevant to practice as an APRN in the specified category;
	• legal, ethical, and professional responsibilities of the APRN; and
	• supervised clinical practice relevant to the specialty of APRN
	5) The curriculum meets the following criteria:
	• Curriculum is consistent with competencies of the specific areas of practice
	• Instructional track/major has a minimum of 500 supervised clinical hours overall
	• The supervised clinical experience is directly related to the knowledge and role of the specialty and category
	C. All individuals, without exception, seeking a national certification must complete a formal didactic and clinical advanced practice program meeting the above criteria.
IV. The standard methodologies used are acceptable to the testing community such as incumbent job analysis study, logical job analysis studies.	A. Exam content based on a job/task analysis. B. Job analysis studies are conducted at least every five years. C. The results of the job analysis study are published and available to the public. D. There is evidence of the content validity of the job analysis study.

V. The examination represents entry-level practice in the advanced nursing practice category.	A. Entry-level practice in the advanced practice specialty is described including the following:
	   1) Process
	   2) Frequency
	   3) Qualifications of the group making the determination
	   4) Geographic representation
	   5) Professional or regulatory organizations involved in the reviews

VI. The examination represents the knowledge, skills, and abilities essential for the delivery of safe and effective advanced nursing care to the clients.	A. The job analysis includes activities representing knowledge, skills, and abilities necessary for competent performance. B. The examination reflects the results of the job analysis study. C. Knowledge, skills, and abilities, which are critical to public safety, are identified. D. The examination content is oriented to educational curriculum practice requirements and accepted standards of care.
VII. Examination items are reviewed for content validity, cultural bias, and correct scoring using an established mechanism, both before use and periodically.	A. Each item is associated with a single cell of the test plan. B. Items are reviewed for currency before each use at least every three years. C. Items are reviewed by members of under-represented gender and ethnicities who are active in the field being certified. Reviewers have been trained to distinguish irrelevant cultural dependencies from knowledge necessary to safe and effective practice. Process for identifying and processing flagged items is identified.

26

APRN Joint Dialogue Group Report, July 7, 2008

	D. A statistical bias analysis is performed on all items.
	E. All items are subjected to an "unscored" use for data collection purposes before their first use as a "scored" item.
	F. A process to detect and eliminate bias from the test is in place.
	G. Reuse guidelines for items on an exam form are identified.
	H. Item writing and review is done by qualified individuals who represent specialties, population subgroups, etc.
VIII. Examinations are evaluated for psychometric performance.	A. Reference groups used for comparative analysis are defined.
IX. The passing standard is established using acceptable psychometric methods, and is re-evaluated periodically.	A. Passing standard is criterion-referenced.
X. Examination security is maintained through established procedures.	A. Protocols are established to maintain security related to: 1) Item development (e.g., item writers and confidentiality, how often items are re-used) 2) Maintenance of question pool 3) Printing and production process 4) Storage and transportation of examination is secure 5) Administration of examination (e.g., who administers, who checks administrators) 6) Ancillary materials (e.g., test keys, scrap materials) 7) Scoring of examination 8) Occurrence of a crisis (e.g., exam is compromised, etc)
XI. Certification is issued based upon passing the examination and meeting all other certification requirements.	A. Certification process is described, including the following: 1) Criteria for certification decisions are identified 2) The verification that passing exam results and all other requirements are met 3) Procedures are in place for appealing decisions B. There is due process for situations such as nurses denied access to the examination or nurses who have had their certification revoked. C. A mechanism is in place for communicating with candidate. D. Confidentiality of nonpublic candidate data is maintained.
XII. A retake policy is in place.	A. Failing candidates permitted to be reexamined at a future date. B. Failing candidates informed of procedures for retakes. C. Test for repeating examinees should be equivalent to the test for first time candidates. D. Repeating examinees should be expected to meet the same test performance standards as first time examinees. E. Failing candidates are given information on content areas of deficiency. F. Repeating examinees are not exposed to the same items when taking the exam previously.
XIII. Certification maintenance	A. Certification maintenance requirements are specified (e.g., continuing

27

APRN Joint Dialogue Group Report, July 7, 2008

program, which includes review of qualifications and continued competence, is in place.	education, practice, examination, etc.).
	B. Certification maintenance procedures include:
	  1) Procedures for ensuring match between continued competency measures and APRN specialty
	  2) Procedures for validating information provided by candidates
	  3) Procedures for issuing re-certification
	C. Professional staff oversee credential review.
	D. Certification maintenance is required a minimum of every 5 years.

XIV. Mechanisms are in place for communication to boards of nursing for timely verification of an individual's certification status, changes in certification status, and changes in the certification program, including qualifications, test plan and scope of practice.	A. Communication mechanisms address:
	  1) Permission obtained from candidates to share information regarding the certification process
	  2) Procedures to provide verification of certification to Boards of Nursing
	  3) Procedures for notifying Boards of Nursing regarding changes of certification status
	  4) Procedures for notification of changes in certification programs (qualifications, test plan or scope of practice) to Boards of Nursing

XV. An evaluation process is in place to provide quality assurance in its certification program.	A. Internal review panels are used to establish quality assurance procedures.
	  1) Composition of these groups (by title or area of expertise) is described
	  2) Procedures are reviewed
	  3) Frequency of review
	B. Procedures are in place to ensure adherence to established QA policy and procedures.

Revised 11-6-01

28

APRN Joint Dialogue Group Report, July 7, 2008

APPENDIX B
American Nurses Association
Congress on Nursing Practice and Economics
2004
Recognition as a Nursing Specialty

The process of recognizing an area of practice as a nursing specialty allows the profession to formally identify subset areas of focused practice. A clear description of that nursing practice assists the larger community of nurses, healthcare consumers, and others to gain familiarity and understanding of the nursing specialty. Therefore, the document requesting ANA recognition must clearly and fully address each of the fourteen specialty recognition criteria. The inclusion of additional materials to support the discussion and promote understanding of the criteria is acceptable. A scope of practice statement must accompany the submission requesting recognition as a nursing specialty.

Criteria for Recognition as a Nursing Specialty

The following criteria are used by the Congress on Nursing Practice and Economics in the review and decision-making processes to recognize an area of practice as a nursing specialty:

A nursing specialty:
1. Defines itself as nursing.

2. Adheres to the overall licensure requirements of the profession.

3. Subscribes to the overall purposes and functions of nursing.

4. Is clearly defined.

5. Is practiced nationally or internationally.

6. Includes a substantial number of nurses who devote most of their practice to the specialty.

7. Can identify a need and demand for itself.

8. Has a well derived knowledge base particular to the practice of the nursing specialty.

9. Is concerned with phenomena of the discipline of nursing.

10. Defines competencies for the area of nursing specialty practice.

11. Has existing mechanisms for supporting, reviewing and disseminating research to support its knowledge base.

12. Has defined educational criteria for specialty preparation or graduate degree.

13. Has continuing education programs or continuing competence mechanisms for nurses in the specialty.

14. Is organized and represented by a national specialty association or branch of a parent organization.

29

APRN Joint Dialogue Group Report, July 7, 2008

APPENDIX C

NCBN APRN Committee Members 2003 -2008

2003
- Katherine Thomas, Executive Director, Texas Board of Nurse Examiners
- Patty Brown, Board Staff, Kansas State Board of Nursing
- Kim Powell, Board President, Montana Board of Nursing
- Charlene Hanson, Consultant
- Georgia Manning, Arkansas State Board of Nursing
- Deborah Bohannon-Johnson, Board President, North Dakota Board of Nursing
- Jane Garvin, Board President, Maryland Board of Nursing
- Janet Younger, Board President, Virginia Board of Nursing
- Nancy Chornick, NCSBN

2004
- Katherine Thomas, Executive Director, Texas Board of Nurse Examiners
- Patty Brown, Board Staff, Kansas State Board of Nursing
- Kim Powell, Board President, Montana Board of Nursing
- Charlene Hanson, Consultant
- Janet Younger, Board President, Virginia Board of Nursing
- Polly Johnson, Board Representative, North Carolina Board of Nursing
- Laura Poe, Member, Utah State Board of Nursing
- Georgia Manning, Arkansas State Board of Nursing
- Jane Garvin RN, Board President, Maryland Board of Nursing
- Ann Forbes, Board Staff, North Carolina Board of Nursing
- Nancy Chornick, NCSBN

2005
- Katherine Thomas, Executive Director, Texas Board of Nurse Examiners
- Patty Brown, Board Staff, Kansas State Board of Nursing
- Charlene Hanson, Consultant
- Janet Younger, Board President, Virginia Board of Nursing
- Polly Johnson, Board Representative, North Carolina Board of Nursing
- Laura Poe, Member, Utah State Board of Nursing
- Marcia Hobbs, Board Member, Kentucky Board of Nursing
- Randall Hudspeth, Board Member, Idaho Board of Nursing
- Ann Forbes, Board Staff, North Carolina Board of Nursing
- Cristiana Rosa, Board Member, Rhode Island Board of Nurse
- Kim Powell, Board President, Montana Board of Nursing
- Nancy Chornick, NCSBN

2006
- Katherine Thomas, Executive Director, Texas Board of Nurse Examiners
- Patty Brown, Board Staff, Kansas State Board of Nursing
- Charlene Hanson, Consultant
- Janet Younger, Board President, Virginia Board of Nursing
- Laura Poe, Member, Utah State Board of Nursing

30

APRN Joint Dialogue Group Report, July 7, 2008

- Marcia Hobbs, Board Member, Kentucky Board of Nursing
- Randall Hudspeth, Board Member, Idaho Board of Nursing
- Cristiana Rosa, Board Member, Rhode Island Board of Nurse
- James Luther Raper, Board Member, Alabama Board of Nursing
- Linda Rice, Board Member, Vermont Board of Nursing
- Cathy Williamson, Board Member, Mississippi Board of Nursing
- Ann Forbes, Board Staff, North Carolina Board of Nursing
- Polly Johnson, Board Representative, North Carolina Board of Nursing
- Sheila N. Kaiser, Board Vice-Chair, Massachusetts Board of Registration in Nursing
- Nancy Chornick, NCSBN

2007
- Faith Fields, Board Liaison, Arkansas State Board of Nursing
- Katherine Thomas, Executive Director, Texas Board of Nurse Examiners
- Ann L. O'Sullivan, Board Member, Pennsylvania Board of Nursing
- Patty Brown, Board Staff, Kansas State Board of Nursing
- Charlene Hanson, Consultant
- Laura Poe, Member, Utah State Board of Nursing
- John C. Preston, Board Member, Tennessee Board of Nursing
- Randall Hudspeth, Board Member, Idaho Board of Nursing
- Cristiana Rosa, Board Member, Rhode Island Board of Nurse
- James Luther Raper, Board Member, Alabama Board of Nursing
- Linda Rice, Board Member, Vermont Board of Nursing
- Cathy Williamson, Board Member, Mississippi Board of Nursing
- Janet Younger, Board President, Virginia Board of Nursing
- Marcia Hobbs, Board Member, Kentucky Board of Nursing
- Nancy Chornick, NCSBN

2008
- Doreen K. Begley, Board Member, Nevada State Board of Nursing
- Ann L. O'Sullivan, Board Member, Pennsylvania Board of Nursing
- Patty Brown, Board Staff, Kansas State Board of Nursing
- Charlene Hanson, Consultant
- Laura Poe, Member, Utah State Board of Nursing
- John C. Preston, Board Member, Tennessee Board of Nursing
- Randall Hudspeth, Board Member, Idaho Board of Nursing
- Cristiana Rosa, Board Member, Rhode Island Board of Nurse
- James Luther Raper, Board Member, Alabama Board of Nursing
- Linda Rice, Board Member, Vermont Board of Nursing
- Cathy Williamson, Board Member, Mississippi Board of Nursing
- Tracy Klein, Member Staff, Oregon State Board of Nursing
- Darlene Byrd, Board Member, Arkansas State Board of Nursing
- Nancy Chornick, NCSBN

31

APRN Joint Dialogue Group Report, July 7, 2008

Appendix D

2006 NCSBN APRN Roundtable
Organization Attendance List

Alabama Board of Nursing

American Academy of Nurse Practitioners

American Academy of Nurse Practitioners National Certification Program, Inc

American Association of Colleges of Nursing

American Association of Critical-Care Nurses

American Association of Nurse Anesthetists

American Association of Psychiatric Nurses

American Board of Nursing Specialties

American College of Nurse Practitioners

American College of Nurse-Midwives

American Holistic Nurses' Certification Corporation

American Midwifery Certification Board

American Nurses Association

American Nurses Credentialing Center

American Organization of Nurses Executives

Association of Women's Health, Obstetric and Neonatal Nurses

Board of Certification for Emergency Nursing

Council on Accreditation of Nurse Anesthesia Educational Programs

Emergency Nurses Association

George Washington School of Medicine

Idaho Board of Nursing

Kansas Board of Nursing

Kentucky Board of Nursing

Massachusetts Board of Nursing

Mississippi Board of Nursing

National Association of Clinical Nurse Specialists

National Association of Nurse Practitioners in Women's Health

National Association of Pediatric Nurse Practitioners

National Board for Certification of Hospice & Palliative Nurses

National Certification Corporation for the Obstetric, Gynecologic and Neonatal Nursing Specialties

National League for Nursing Accrediting Commission

32

APRN Joint Dialogue Group Report, July 7, 2008

North Carolina Board of Nursing

Oncology Nursing Certification Corporation

Pediatric Nursing Certification Board

Rhode Island Board of Nursing

Texas Board of Nurse Examiners

Utah Board of Nursing

Vermont Board of Nursing

Wound, Ostomy and Continence Nursing Certification Board

2007 APRN Roundtable Attendance List

American Association of Colleges of Nursing

ABNS Accreditation Council

Alabama Board of Nursing

American Academy of Nurse Practitioners

American Academy of Nurse Practitioners National Certification Program, Inc

American Association of Critical-Care Nurses

American Association of Nurse Anesthetists

American College of Nurse-Midwives

American College of Nurse Practitioners

American Midwifery Certification Board

American Nurses Credentialing Center - Certification Services

American Organization of Nurse Executives

Arkansas State Board of Nursing

Association of Women's Health, Obstetric and Neonatal Nurses

Board of Certification for Emergency Nursing

Colorado Board of Nursing

Commission on Collegiate Nursing Education

Council on Accreditation of Nurse Anesthesia Educational Programs

Council on Certification of Nurse Anesthetists and Council on Recertification of Nurse Anesthetists

Emergency Nurses Association

Idaho Board of Nursing

Illinois State Board of Nursing

Kansas Board of Nursing

Kentucky Board of Nursing

33

APRN Joint Dialogue Group Report, July 7, 2008

Loyola University Chicago Niehoff School of Nursing

Minnesota Board of Nursing

Mississippi Board of Nursing

National Association of Clinical Nurse Specialists

National Association of Pediatric Nurse Practitioners

National League for Nursing Accrediting Commission

National Organization of Nurse Practitioner Faculties

National Certification Corporation for the Obstetric, Gynecologic and Neonatal Nursing Specialties

Oncology Nursing Certification Corporation

Pennsylvania Board of Nursing

Pediatric Nursing Certification Board

Rhode Island Board of Nursing

Rush University College of Nursing

South Dakota Board of Nursing

Tennessee Board of Nursing

Texas Board of Nurse Examiners

Vermont Board of Nursing

34

APRN Joint Dialogue Group Report, July 7, 2008

APPENDIX E

APRN Joint Dialogue Group
Organizations represented at the Joint Dialogue Group Meetings

American Academy of Nurse Practitioners Certification Program
American Association of Colleges of Nursing
American Association of Nurse Anesthetists
American College of Nurse-Midwives
American Nurses Association
American Organization of Nurse Executives
Compact Administrators
National Association of Clinical Nurse Specialists
National League for Nursing Accrediting Commission
National Organization of Nurse Practitioner Faculties
National Council of State Boards of Nursing
NCSBN APRN Advisory Committee Representatives (5)

35

APRN Joint Dialogue Group Report, July 7, 2008

Appendix F

**ORGANIZATIONS INVITED TO APN CONSENSUS CONFERENCE
JUNE, 2004**

Accreditation Commission for Midwifery Education
American Academy of Nurse Practitioners
American Academy of Nurse Practitioners Certification Program
American Academy of Nursing
American Association of Critical Care Nurses
American Association of Critical Care Nurses Certification Program
American Association of Nurse Anesthetists
American Association of Occupational Health Nurses
American Board of Nursing Specialties
American College of Nurse Practitioners
American College of Nurse-Midwives
American Nurses Association
American Nurses Credentialing Center
American Organization of Nurse Executives
American Psychiatric Nurses Association
Association of Faculties of Pediatric Nurse Practitioners
Association of Rehabilitation Nurses
Association of Women's Health, Obstetric and Neonatal Nurses
Certification Board Perioperative Nursing
Commission on Collegiate Nursing Education
Council on Accreditation of Nurse Anesthesia Educational Programs
Division of Nursing, DHHS, HRSA
Emergency Nurses Association
Hospice and Palliative Nurses Association
International Nurses Society on Addictions
International Society of Psychiatric-Mental Health Nurses
NANDA International
National Association of Clinical Nurse Specialists
National Association of Neonatal Nurses
National Association of Nurse Practitioners in Women's Health
National Association of Nurse Practitioners in Women's Health, Council on Accreditation
National Association of Pediatric Nurse Practitioners
National Association of School Nurses
National Board for Certification of Hospice and Palliative Nurses
National Certification Corporation for the Obstetric, Gynecologic and Neonatal Nursing
Specialties
National Conference of Gerontological Nurse Practitioners
National Council of State Boards of Nursing
National Gerontological Nursing Association
National League for Nursing
National League for Nursing Accrediting Commission
National Organization of Nurse Practitioner Faculties

36

APRN Joint Dialogue Group Report, July 7, 2008

Nurse Licensure Compact Administrators/State of Utah Department of Commerce/Division
of Occupational & Professional Licensing
Nurses Organization of Veterans Affairs
Oncology Nursing Certification Corporation
Oncology Nursing Society
Pediatric Nursing Certification Board
Sigma Theta Tau, International
Society of Pediatric Nurses
Wound Ostomy & Continence Nurses Society
Wound Ostomy Continence Nursing Certification Board

37

APRN Joint Dialogue Group Report, July 7, 2008

APPENDIX G

ORGANIZATIONS PARTICIPATING IN APRN CONSENSUS PROCESS

Academy of Medical-Surgical Nurses
Accreditation Commission for Midwifery Education
American College of Nurse-midwives Division of Accreditation
American Academy of Nurse Practitioners
American Academy of Nurse Practitioners Certification Program
American Association of Colleges of Nursing
American Association of Critical Care Nurses Certification
American Association of Neuroscience Nurses
American Association of Nurse Anesthetists
American Association of Occupational Health Nurses
American Board for Occupational Health Nurses
American Board of Nursing Specialties
American College of Nurse-Midwives
American College of Nurse Practitioners
American Holistic Nurses Association
American Nephrology Nurses Association
American Nurses Association
American Nurses Credentialing Center
American Organization of Nurse Executives
American Psychiatric Nurses Association
American Society of PeriAnesthesia Nurses
American Society for Pain Management Nursing
Association of Community Health Nursing Educators
Association of Faculties of Pediatric Nurse Practitioners
Association of Nurses in AIDS Care
Association of PeriOperative Registered Nurses
Association of Rehabilitation Nurses
Association of State and Territorial Directors of nursing
Association of Women's Health, Obstetric and Neonatal Nurses
Board of Certification for Emergency Nursing
Council on Accreditation of Nurse Anesthesia Educational Programs
Commission on Collegiate Nursing Education
Commission on Graduates of Foreign Nursing Schools
District of Columbia Board of Nursing
Department of Health
Dermatology Nurses Association
Division of Nursing, DHHS, HRSA
Emergency Nurses Association
George Washington University
Health Resources and Services Administration
Infusion Nurses Society
International Nurses Society on Addictions
International Society of Psychiatric-Mental Health Nurses
Kentucky Board of Nursing

38

APRN Joint Dialogue Group Report, July 7, 2008

National Association of Clinical Nurse Specialists
National Association of Neonatal Nurses
National Association of Nurse Practitioners in Women's Health, Council on Accreditation
National Association of Pediatric Nurse Practitioners
National Association of School of Nurses
National Association of Orthopedic Nurses
National Certification Corporation for the Obstetric, Gynecologic, and Neonatal Nursing Specialties
National Conference of Gerontological Nurse Practitioners
National Council of State Boards of Nursing
National League for Nursing
National League for Nursing Accrediting Commission
National Organization of Nurse Practitioner Faculties
Nephrology Nursing Certification Commission
North American Nursing Diagnosis Association International
Nurses Organization of Veterans Affairs
Oncology Nursing Certification Corporation
Oncology Nursing Society
Pediatric Nursing Certification Board
Pennsylvania State Board of Nursing
Public Health Nursing Section of the American Public Health Association.
Rehabilitation Nursing Certification Board
Society for Vascular Nursing
Texas Nurses Association
Texas State Board of Nursing
Utah State Board of Nursing
Women's Health, Obstetric & Neonatal Nurses
Wound, Ostomy, & Continence Nurses Society
Wound, Ostomy, & Continence Nursing Certification

39

APRN Joint Dialogue Group Report, July 7, 2008

APPENDIX H

APRN CONSENSUS PROCESS WORK GROUP
ORGANIZATIONS THAT WERE REPRESENTED AT THE WORK GROUP MEETINGS

Jan Towers, American Academy of Nurse Practitioners Certification Program
Joan Stanley, American Association of Colleges of Nursing
Carol Hartigan, American Association of Critical Care Nurses Certification Corporation
Leo LeBel, American Association of Nurse Anesthetists
Bonnie Niebuhr, American Board of Nursing Specialties
Peter Johnson & Elaine Germano, American College of Nurse-Midwives
Mary Jean Schumann, American Nurses Association
Mary Smolenski, American Nurses Credentialing Center
M.T. Meadows, American Organization of Nurse Executives
Edna Hamera & Sandra Talley, American Psychiatric Nurses Association
Elizabeth Hawkins-Walsh, Association of Faculties of Pediatric Nurse Practitioners
Jennifer Butlin, Commission on Collegiate Nursing Education
Laura Poe, APRN Compact Administrators
Betty Horton, Council on Accreditation of Nurse Anesthesia Educational Programs
Kelly Goudreau, National Association of Clinical Nurse Specialists
Fran Way, National Association of Nurse Practitioners in Women's Health, Council on
Accreditation
Mimi Bennett, National Certification Corporation for the Obstetric, Gynecologic, and
Neonatal Nursing Specialties
Kathy Apple, National Council of State Boards of Nursing
Grace Newsome & Sharon Tanner, National League for Nursing Accrediting Commission
Kitty Werner & Ann O'Sullivan, National Organization of Nurse Practitioner Faculties
Cyndi Miller-Murphy, Oncology Nursing Certification Corporation
Janet Wyatt, Pediatric Nursing Certification Board
Carol Calianno, Wound, Ostomy and Continence Nursing Certification Board
Irene Sandvold, DHHS, HRSA, Division of Nursing *(observer)*

40

APRN Joint Dialogue Group Report, July 7, 2008

ADDENDUM

Example of a National Consensus-Building Process to Develop Nationally Recognized Education Standards and Role/Specialty Competencies

The national consensus-based process described here was originally designed, with funding by the Department of Health and Human Services, Health Resources and Services Administration, Bureau of Health Professions, Division of Nursing, to develop and validate national consensus-based primary care nurse practitioner competencies in five specialty areas. The process was developed with consultation from a nationally recognized expert in higher education assessment. The process subsequently has been used and validated for the development of similar sets of competencies for other areas of nursing practice, including competencies for mass casualty education for all nurses and competencies for acute care nurse practitioners and psych/mental health nurse practitioners.

This process for developing nationally recognized educational standards, nationally recognized role competencies and nationally recognized specialty competencies is an iterative, step-wise process. The steps are:

Step 1: At the request of the organization(s) representing the role or specialty, a neutral group or groups convenes and facilitates a national panel of all stakeholder organizations as defined in step 2.

Step 2: To ensure broad representation, invitations to participate should be extended to one representative of each of the recognized nursing accrediting organizations, certifiers within the role and specialty, groups whose primary mission is graduate education and who have established educational criteria for the identified role and specialty, and groups with competencies and standards for education programs that prepare individuals in the role and specialty.

Step 3: Organizational representatives serving on the national consensus panel bring and share role delineation studies, competencies for practice and education, scopes and standards of practice, and standards for education programs.

Step 4: Agreement is reached among the panel members

Step 5: Panel members take the draft to their individual boards for feedback.

Step 6: That feedback is returned to the panel. This is an iterative process until agreement is reached.

Step 7: Validation is sought from a larger group of stakeholders including organizations and individuals. This is known as the Validation Panel.

Step 8: Feedback from the Validation Panel is returned to National Panel to prepare the final document.

Step 9: Final document is sent to boards represented on the National Panel and the Validation Panel for endorsement.

The final document demonstrates national consensus through consideration of broad input from key stakeholders. The document is then widely disseminated.

41

Appendix B.

Nursing's Social Policy Statement, 2nd Edition (2003)

The content in this appendix is not current and is of historical significance only.

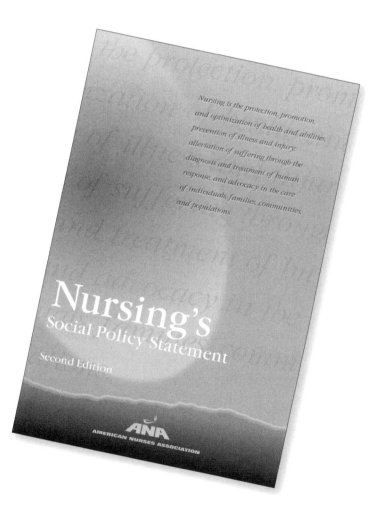

INTRODUCTION

"Nursing is the pivotal health care profession, highly valued for its specialized knowledge, skill and caring in improving the health status of the public and ensuring safe, effective, quality care. The profession mirrors the diverse population it serves and provides leadership to create positive changes in health policy and delivery systems. Individuals choose nursing as a career, and remain in the profession, because of the opportunities for personal and professional growth, supportive work environments and compensation commensurate with roles and responsibilities.[1]

The Social Context of Nursing

Nursing's Social Policy Statement, Second Edition expresses the social contract between society and the profession of nursing. Registered nurses and others can use this document as a framework for understanding professional nursing's relationship with society and its obligation to those who receive professional nursing care. It includes a definition of professional nursing, descriptions of professional nursing and its knowledge base, and brief descriptions of the scope of professional nursing practice and the methods by which the profession is regulated. These concepts underlie the practice of professional nursing, provide direction for clinicians, educators, administrators, and scientists within professional nursing, and inform other healthcare professionals, public policymakers, and funding bodies about professional nursing's contribution to health care.

This statement is derived from the 1980 landmark document, *Nursing: A Social Policy Statement,*[2] and *Nursing's Social Policy Statement,*[3] published in 1995. These documents provided the profession's earlier descriptions of its social responsibility and professional nursing's roles in the American healthcare system. The current document presents the practice of professional nursing as it has evolved, and provides direction for the future.

Professional nursing, like other professions, is an essential part of the society from which it grew and within which it continues to evolve. Professional nursing is dynamic, rather than static, reflecting the changing nature of societal needs. Professional nursing can be said to be owned by society, in the sense that "a profession acquires recognition, relevance, and

1

even meaning in terms of its relationship to that society, its culture and institutions, and its other members."[4] This social contract between the broader society and its professions has been expressed as follows:

> Societies (and often vested interests within them)… determine, in accord with their different technological and economic levels of development and their socioeconomic, political and cultural conditions and values, what professional skills and knowledge they most need or desire… Logically, then, the professions open to individuals in any particular society are the property not of the individual but of the society. What individuals acquire through training is professional knowledge and skill, not a profession or even part ownership of one.[5]

The authority for the practice of professional nursing is based on a social contract that acknowledges professional rights and responsibilities as well as mechanisms for public accountability.

> Society grants the professions authority over functions vital to itself and permits them considerable autonomy in the conduct of their affairs. In return, the professions are expected to act responsibly, always mindful of the public trust. Self-regulation to assure quality in performance is at the heart of this relationship. It is the authentic hallmark of a mature profession.[6]

To maximize the contributions nurses make to society, it is necessary to protect the dignity and autonomy of nurses in the workplace. To that end, the American Nurses Association has adopted the *Bill of Rights for Registered Nurses.*[7]

2   *Nursing's Social Policy Statement: Second Edition*

Values and Assumptions of Nursing's Social Contract

The following values and assumptions undergird professional nursing's contract with society:

- Humans manifest an essential unity of mind, body, and spirit.

- Human experience is contextually and culturally defined.

- Health and illness are human experiences. The presence of illness does not preclude health nor does optimal health preclude illness.

- The relationship between nurse and patient involves participation of both in the process of care.

- The interaction between nurse and patient occurs within the context of the values and beliefs of the patient and the nurse.

- Public policy and the healthcare delivery system influence the health and well-being of society and professional nursing.

These values and assumptions apply whether the recipient of professional nursing care is an individual, family, group, community, or population.

Introduction   3

DEFINITION OF NURSING

Definitions of nursing have evolved to acknowledge six essential features of professional nursing:

- provision of a caring relationship that facilitates health and healing,

- attention to the range of human experiences and responses to health and illness within the physical and social environments,

- integration of objective data with knowledge gained from an appreciation of the patient or group's subjective experience,

- application of scientific knowledge to the processes of diagnosis and treatment through the use of judgment and critical thinking,

- advancement of professional nursing knowledge through scholarly inquiry, and

- influence on social and public policy to promote social justice.

In her *Notes on Nursing: What It Is and What It Is Not*, published in 1859, Florence Nightingale defined nursing as having "charge of the personal health of somebody...and what nursing has to do...is to put the patient in the best condition for nature to act upon him."[8]

A century later, Virginia Henderson defined the purpose of nursing as "to assist the individual, sick or well, in the performance of those activities contributing to health or its recovery (or to a peaceful death) that he would perform unaided if he had the necessary strength, will or knowledge. And to do this in such a way as to help him gain independence as rapidly as possible."[9]

In the 1980 *Nursing: A Social Policy Statement*, nursing was defined as "the diagnosis and treatment of human responses to actual or potential health problems."[10]

5

A broader definition is consistent with professional nursing's commitment to meeting societal needs, and permits the profession and its practitioners to adapt to the ongoing changes in healthcare environments, practice expectations, and the profession itself. The evolution of nursing practice leads to the following definition of professional nursing:

Nursing is the protection, promotion, and optimization of health and abilities, prevention of illness and injury, alleviation of suffering through the diagnosis and treatment of human response, and advocacy in the care of individuals, families, communities, and populations.[1]

Moreover, nursing addresses the organizational, social, economic, legal, and political factors within the healthcare system and society. These and other factors affect the cost, access to, and quality of health care and the vitality of the nursing profession. This is accomplished through a variety of means.

KNOWLEDGE BASE FOR NURSING PRACTICE

Nursing is a profession and a scientific discipline. The knowledge base for professional nursing practice includes nursing science, philosophy, and ethics, as well as physical, economic, biomedical, behavioral, and social sciences. To refine and expand the knowledge base and science of the discipline, nurses generate and use theories and research findings that are selected on the basis of their fit with professional nursing's values of health and health care, as well as their relevance to professional nursing practice.

Nurses are concerned with human experiences and responses across the lifespan. Nurses partner with individuals, families, communities, and populations to address issues such as:

- promotion of health and safety;
- care and self-care processes;
- physical, emotional, and spiritual comfort, discomfort, and pain;
- adaptation to physiologic and pathophysiologic processes;
- emotions related to experiences of birth, growth and development, health, illness, disease, and death;
- meanings ascribed to health and illness;
- decision-making and ability to make choices;
- relationships, role performance, and change processes within relationships;
- social policies and their effects on the health of individuals, families, and communities;
- healthcare systems and their relationships with access to and quality of health care; and
- the environment and the prevention of disease.

Nurses use their theoretical and evidence-based knowledge of these phenomena in collaborating with patients to assess, plan, implement, and evaluate care. Nursing interventions are intended to produce beneficial effects and contribute to quality outcomes. Nurses evaluate the effectiveness of their care in relation to identified outcomes and use evidence to improve care.

7

Scope of Nursing Practice

Professional nursing has one scope of practice, which encompasses the range of activities from those of the beginning registered nurse through the advanced level. While a single scope of professional nursing practice exists, the depth and breadth to which individual nurses engage in the total scope of professional nursing practice is dependent on their educational preparation, their experience, their role, and the nature of the patient population they serve.

Further, all nurses are responsible for practicing in accordance with recognized standards of professional nursing practice and professional performance. The level of application of standards varies with the education, experience, and skills of the individual nurse. Since 1965, ANA has consistently affirmed the baccalaureate degree in nursing as the preferred educational requirement for entry into professional nursing practice.[12] Each nurse remains accountable for the quality of care within his or her scope of nursing practice.

Professional nursing's scope of practice is dynamic and continually evolving. It has a flexible boundary that is responsive to the changing needs of society and the expanding knowledge base of its theoretical and scientific domains. This scope of practice thus overlaps those of other professions involved in health care. The boundaries of each profession are constantly changing, and members of various professions cooperate by sharing knowledge, techniques, and ideas about how to deliver quality health care. Collaboration among healthcare professionals involves recognition of the expertise of others within and outside the profession, and referral to those other providers when appropriate. Collaboration also involves some shared functions and a common focus on the same overall mission.

Nurses provide care for patients in a variety of settings. Nurses may initiate treatments or carry out interventions initiated by other authorized healthcare providers. Nurses are coordinators of care as well as caregivers.

Nursing practice includes, but is not limited to, initiating and maintaining comfort measures, promoting and supporting human functions and responses, establishing an environment conducive to well-being, providing health counseling and teaching, and collaborating on certain aspects of the health regimen. This practice is based on understanding the human condition across the life span and the relationship of the individual within the environment.

8   *Nursing's Social Policy Statement: Second Edition*

Nursing care is provided and directed by registered nurses and advanced practice registered nurses. All registered nurses are educated in the art and science of nursing with the goal of helping patients to attain, maintain, and restore health, or to experience a dignified death. Registered nurses and advanced practice registered nurses may also develop expertise in a particular specialty.

Specialization in Nursing

Specialization involves focusing on a part of the whole field of professional nursing. The American Nurses Association and specialty nursing organizations delineate the components of professional nursing practice that are essential for any particular specialty. Registered nurses may seek certification in a variety of specialized areas of nursing practice.

Advanced Practice Registered Nurses

Advanced practice registered nurses (that is, nurse practitioners, certified registered nurse anesthetists, certified nurse-midwives, and clinical nurse specialists) practice from both *expanded* and *specialized* knowledge and skills.

- *Expansion* refers to the acquisition of new practice knowledge and skills, including the knowledge and skills that authorize role autonomy within areas of practice that may overlap traditional boundaries of medical practice.

- *Specialization* is concentrating or delimiting one's focus to part of the whole field of professional nursing (such as ambulatory care, pediatric, maternal-child, psychiatric, palliative care, or oncology nursing).

Advanced practice is characterized by the integration and application of a broad range of theoretical and evidence-based knowledge that occurs as a part of graduate nursing education. Advanced practice registered nurses hold master's or doctoral degrees and are licensed, certified, and/or approved to practice in their roles.

Knowledge Base for Nursing Practice   9

Additional Advanced Roles

Continuation of the profession of nursing is also dependent on the education of nurses, appropriate organization of nursing services, continued expansion of nursing knowledge, and the development and adoption of policies consistent with values and assumptions that underlie the scope of professional nursing practice. Registered nurses may practice in such advanced roles as nurse educator, nurse administrator, nurse researcher, and nurse policy analyst. These advanced roles require specific additional knowledge and skills at the graduate level. Generally, those practicing in these roles hold master's or doctoral degrees.

Further details on the scope of professional nursing practice, specifics describing the *who, what, where, when, why,* and *how* of both specialized and advanced areas of nursing practice, are found in the current version of *Nursing: Scope and Standards of Practice.*[13]

10   *Nursing's Social Policy Statement: Second Edition*

THE REGULATION OF NURSING PRACTICE

Professional nursing, like other professions, is accountable for ensuring that its members act in the public interest in the course of providing the unique service society has entrusted to them. The processes by which the profession does this include self-regulation, professional regulation, and legal regulation.

Self-Regulation

Self-regulation involves personal accountability for the knowledge base for professional practice. Nurses develop and maintain current knowledge, skills, and abilities through formal and continuing education. Where appropriate, nurses hold certification in their area of practice to demonstrate this accountability.

Nurses also regulate themselves as individuals through peer review of their practice. Continuous performance improvement fosters the refinement of knowledge, skills, and clinical decision-making processes at all levels and in all areas of professional nursing practice. As expressed in the profession's code of ethics, peer review is one mechanism by which nurses are held accountable for practice

As noted in Provision 3.4 (Standards and Review Mechanisms) of *Code of Ethics for Nurses with Interpretive Statements*,[14] nurses should also be active participants in the development of policies and review mechanisms designed to promote patient safety, reduce the likelihood of errors, and address both environmental system factors and human factors that present increased risk to patients. In addition, when errors do occur, nurses are expected to follow established guidelines in reporting errors committed or observed.

11

Professional Regulation

Professional nursing defines its practice base, provides for research and development of that practice base, establishes a system for nursing education, establishes the structures through which nursing services will be delivered, and provides quality review mechanisms such as a code of ethics, standards of practice, structures for peer review, and a system of credentialing.

Professional regulation of nursing practice begins with the profession's definition of nursing and the scope of professional nursing practice. Professional standards are then derived from the scope of professional nursing practice.

Certification is a judgment of competence made by nurses who are themselves practicing within the area of specialization. Several credentialing boards are associated with the American Nurses Association and with specialty nursing organizations. These boards develop and implement certification examinations and procedures for nurses who wish to have their specialty practice knowledge recognized by the profession and the public. One component of the required evidence is successful completion of an examination that tests the knowledge base for the selected area of practice. Other requirements relate to the content of coursework and amount of supervised practice.

Legal Regulation

All nurses are legally accountable for actions taken in the course of professional nursing practice as well as for actions assigned by the nurse to others assisting in the provision of nursing care. Such accountability is accomplished through the legal regulatory mechanisms of licensure and criminal and civil laws.

The legal contract between society and the professions is defined by statute and by associated rules and regulations. State nurse practice acts and related legislative and regulatory initiatives serve as the explicit codification of the profession's obligation to act in the best interests of society. Nurse practice acts grant nurses the authority to practice and grant society the authority to sanction nurses who violate the norms of the profession or act in a manner that threatens the safety of the public.

Statutory definitions of nursing should be compatible with and build upon the profession's definition of its practice base, but be general enough to provide for the dynamic nature of an evolving scope of nursing practice. Society is best served when consistent definitions of the scope of nursing practice are used by states. This allows residents of all states to access the full range of nursing services.

The Regulation of Nursing Practice   13

CONCLUSION

Nursing's Social Policy Statement, Second Edition describes professional nursing in the United States of America. It includes an identification of the values and the social responsibility of the profession, a definition of professional nursing, a brief discussion of the scope of practice, and a description of professional nursing's knowledge base and the methods by which professional nursing is regulated. *Nursing's Social Policy Statement, Second Edition* provides both an accounting of nursing's professional stewardship and an expression of professional nursing's continuing commitment to the society it serves.

REFERENCES

1. Nursing's Agenda for the Future Steering Committee. *Nursing's Agenda for the Future* (Washington, D.C.: American Nurses Publishing, 2001). Also available on the ANA web site: http://www.nursingworld.org/naf/

2. American Nurses Association. *Nursing: A Social Policy Statement* (Kansas City, MO. American Nurses Association, 1980).

3. American Nurses Association. *Nursing's Social Policy Statement* (Washington, D.C.: American Nurses Publishing, 1995).

4. Page, B.B. "Who owns the profession?," *Hastings Center Report* 5(5): 7–8 (1975).

5. Ibid., 7.

6. Donabedian, A. Foreword in M. Phaneuf, *The Nursing Audit: Self-Regulation in Nursing Practice*, 2nd ed. (New York: Appleton-Century-Crofts, 1972), 8.

7. American Nurses Association. *Bill of Rights for Registered Nurses* (Washington, D.C.: American Nurses Publishing, 2001), 1.

8. Nightingale, F. *Notes on Nursing: What It Is and What It Is Not.* (1859; reprint, New York: J. B. Lippincott Company, 1946), preface, 75.

9. Henderson, V. *Basic Principles of Nursing Care* (London: International Council of Nurses, 1961), 42.

10. American Nurses Association, *Nursing: A Social Policy Statement.* (Kansas City, MO. American Nurses Association, 1980).

11. Adapted from: American Nurses Association. *Code of Ethics for Nurses with Interpretive Statements* (Washington, D.C.: American Nurses Publishing, 2001), 5. (Also on the ANA web site: http://nursingworld.org/ethics/ecode.htm)

12. American Nurses Association House of Delegates. *Titling for Licensure* (Kansas City, MO: American Nurses Association, 1985).

13. American Nurses Association. *Nursing: Scope and Standards of Practice* (Washington, D.C.: American Nurses Publishing, 2003).

14. American Nurses Association, *Code of Ethics for Nurses with Interpretive Statements*, 13–14.

15. Ibid., 24.

15

APPENDIX A
THE DEVELOPMENT OF NURSING'S SOCIAL POLICY STATEMENTS, 1980–2003

Contributors, 1980–2003

Nursing's Social Policy Statement Revision Task Force, 2001–2003
Naomi E. Ervin, RN, PhD, APRN, BC, FAAN; *Chair (2002–2003)*
Anne M. McNamara, PhD, RN; *Chair (2001–2002)*
Linda A. Beechinor, MS, RN, FNP
Joan M. Caley, RN, MS, CNAA, CS
Mary B. Killeen, PhD, RN, C, CNAA
Linda L. Olson, PhD, RN, CNAA
Susan Foley Pierce, PhD, RN
Steven R. Pitkin, RN, MN
Betty Smith-Campbell, PhD, RN, ARNP
Susan Tullai-McGuinness, PhD, MPA, RN
Marva Wade, RN

Social Policy Statement Task Force, 1992–1995
Linda R. Cronenwett, PhD, RN, FAAN; *Facilitator (1994–1995)*
Barbara E. Pokorny, MSN, RN, CS; *Facilitator (1992–1993)*
Kathryn Barnard, PhD, RN, FAAN
Susan E. Doughty, MSN, RN, CS
Beverly Hall, PhD, RN, FAAN
Gail A. Harkness, DrPH, RN, FAAN
Mary S. Koithan, PhD, RN
Frank R. Lamendola, MSN, RN, CS
Mary K. Walker, PhD, RN, FAAN

Nursing: A Social Policy Statement, Authors, 1980
Norma Lang, PhD, RN, FAAN; *Chair*
Nina T. Argondizzo, MA, RN
Kathryn Barnard, PhD, RN, FAAN
Hildegard E. Peplau, EdD, RN, FAAN
Maria C. Phaneuf, MA, RN, FAAN
Jean E. Steel, PhD, RN, FAAN
Glenn Webster, PhD

17

Congress on Nursing Practice and Economics 2002–2004
Anne M. Hammes, MS, RN, CNAA; *Chair*
Marva Wade, RN, *Vice Chair*
Kathryn Ballou, PhD, RN
Joan M. Caley, MS, RN, CS, CNAA
Naomi E. Ervin, RN, PhD, APRN, BC, FAAN
Tracy A. Hollar-Ruegg, MS, RN, CNP
Saul Josman, MN, RN, APRN-BC
David Marshall, JD, RN, CNAA
Mary A. Maryland, PhD, APRN,BC , APN
Maureen Ann Nalle, PhD, RN
Susan Foley Pierce, PhD, RN
Steven R. Pitkin, RN, MN
Lorna Samuels, BSN, RN, BC
Cathalene Teahan, MSN, RN, CNS
Susan Tullai-McGuinness, PhD, MPA, RN

Congress on Nursing Practice and Economics 2000–2002
Linda J. Gobis, JD, RN, FNP; *Chair*
Anne M. McNamara, PhD, RN, *Vice Chair*
Linda A. Beechinor, MS, RN, FNP
Sharon Bidwell-Cerone, PhD, RN, CS-PNP
Joan M. Caley, RN, MS, CNAA, CS
Mary Chaffee, MS, RN, CNA, CCRN
Naomi E. Ervin, PhD, RN, CS, FAAN
Anne M. Hammes, MS, RN, CNAA
Saul Josman, MN, RN, APRN-BC
Mary B. Killeen, PhD, RN, C, CNAA
Patricia (Patti) J. Kummeth, MSN, RN, C
David Marshall, JD RN, BSN
Linda L. Olson, PhD, RN, CNAA
Steven R. Pitkin, RN, MN
Lorna Samuels, BSN, RN, C
Marva Wade, RN

18   *Nursing's Social Policy Statement: Second Edition*

Appendix C.

Nursing's Social Policy Statement (1995)

The content in this appendix is not current and is of historical significance only.

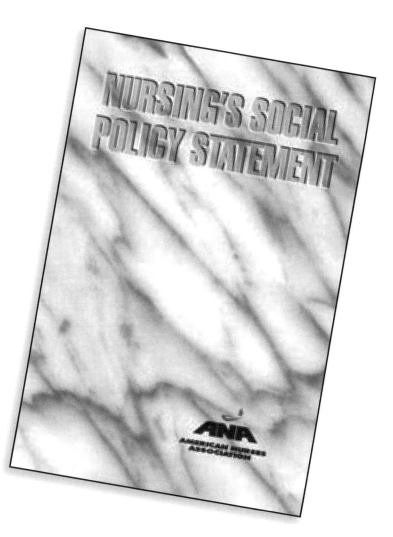

CONTENTS

PREFACE

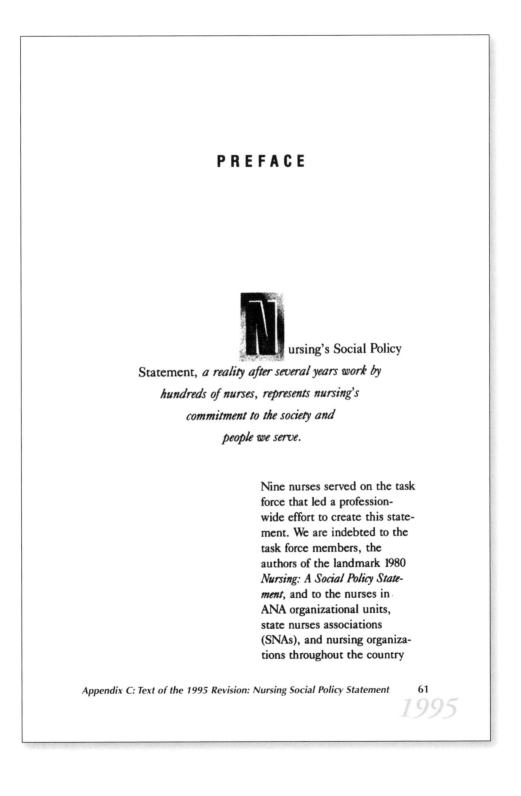

ursing's Social Policy Statement, *a reality after several years work by hundreds of nurses, represents nursing's commitment to the society and people we serve.*

Nine nurses served on the task force that led a profession-wide effort to create this statement. We are indebted to the task force members, the authors of the landmark 1980 *Nursing: A Social Policy Statement*, and to the nurses in ANA organizational units, state nurses associations (SNAs), and nursing organizations throughout the country

Appendix C: Text of the 1995 Revision: Nursing Social Policy Statement 61

1995

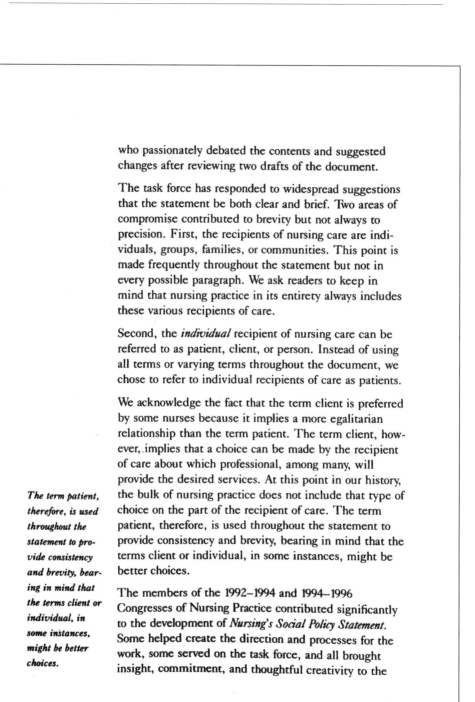

who passionately debated the contents and suggested changes after reviewing two drafts of the document.

The task force has responded to widespread suggestions that the statement be both clear and brief. Two areas of compromise contributed to brevity but not always to precision. First, the recipients of nursing care are individuals, groups, families, or communities. This point is made frequently throughout the statement but not in every possible paragraph. We ask readers to keep in mind that nursing practice in its entirety always includes these various recipients of care.

Second, the *individual* recipient of nursing care can be referred to as patient, client, or person. Instead of using all terms or varying terms throughout the document, we chose to refer to individual recipients of care as patients.

We acknowledge the fact that the term client is preferred by some nurses because it implies a more egalitarian relationship than the term patient. The term client, however, implies that a choice can be made by the recipient of care about which professional, among many, will provide the desired services. At this point in our history, the bulk of nursing practice does not include that type of choice on the part of the recipient of care. The term patient, therefore, is used throughout the statement to provide consistency and brevity, bearing in mind that the terms client or individual, in some instances, might be better choices.

The term patient, therefore, is used throughout the statement to provide consistency and brevity, bearing in mind that the terms client or individual, in some instances, might be better choices.

The members of the 1992–1994 and 1994–1996 Congresses of Nursing Practice contributed significantly to the development of *Nursing's Social Policy Statement*. Some helped create the direction and processes for the work, some served on the task force, and all brought insight, commitment, and thoughtful creativity to the

62

Nursing's Social Policy Statement: Second Edition

1995

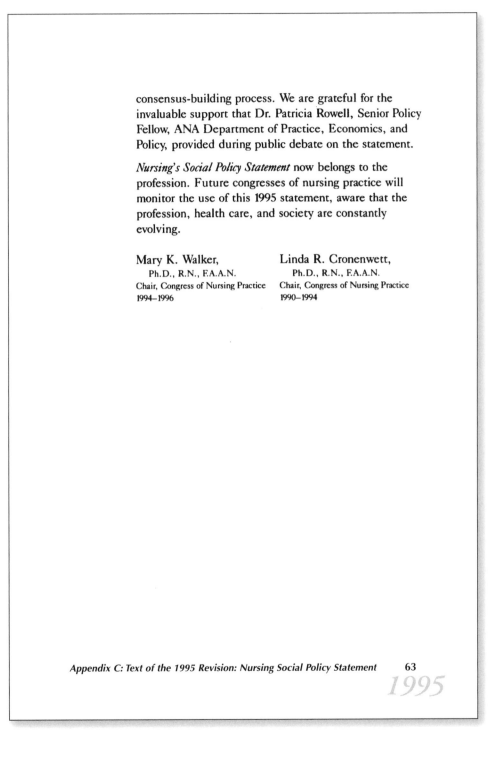

consensus-building process. We are grateful for the invaluable support that Dr. Patricia Rowell, Senior Policy Fellow, ANA Department of Practice, Economics, and Policy, provided during public debate on the statement.

Nursing's Social Policy Statement now belongs to the profession. Future congresses of nursing practice will monitor the use of this 1995 statement, aware that the profession, health care, and society are constantly evolving.

Mary K. Walker,
Ph.D., R.N., F.A.A.N.
Chair, Congress of Nursing Practice
1994–1996

Linda R. Cronenwett,
Ph.D., R.N., F.A.A.N.
Chair, Congress of Nursing Practice
1990–1994

Appendix C: Text of the 1995 Revision: Nursing Social Policy Statement   63

1995

INTRODUCTION

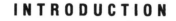 ursing's Social Policy Statement *is a document that nurses can use as a framework for understanding nursing's relationship with society and nursing's obligation to those who receive nursing care.*

The statement includes descriptions of nursing and its knowledge base, the scope of nursing practice, and the methods by which the profession is regulated. The conceptualization of the clinical practice of nursing that is the focus of this statement will provide direction for clinicians,

64

Nursing's Social Policy Statement: Second Edition

1995

educators, administrators, and scientists within the profession of nursing and inform other health care professionals, public policy makers, and funding entities about nursing's contribution to health care.

This statement is derived from the landmark document, *Nursing: A Social Policy Statement* (1980),[1] the profession's first description of its social responsibility and nursing's roles in the American health care system. The current document presents clinical nursing practice as it has evolved according to society's health needs and sets direction for the future.

The Social Context of Nursing

Nursing, like other professions, is an essential part of the society from which it has grown and within which it continues to evolve. Nursing is dynamic, rather than static, and reflects the changing nature of societal need. Nursing can be said to be "owned by society" in the sense that "a profession acquires recognition, relevance, and even meaning in terms of its relationship to that society, its culture and institutions, and its other members."[2]

This social contract between the broader society and its professions has been expressed as follows:

> "Professions acquire recognition and relevance primarily in terms of needs, conditions, and traditions of particular societies and their members . . . societies (and often vested interests within them) . . . determine, in accord with their different technological and economic levels of development and their socioeconomic, political, and cultural conditions and values, what professional skills and knowledge they most need and desire. . . .

Appendix C: Text of the 1995 Revision: Nursing Social Policy Statement   65

1995

The authority for the practice of nursing is based on a social contract that acknowledges professional rights and responsibilities as well as mechanisms for public accountability.

"Logically, then, the professions open to individuals in any particular society are the property not of the individual but of society. What individuals acquire through training is professional knowledge and skill, not a profession or even part ownership of one."[2]

The authority for the practice of nursing is based on a social contract that acknowledges professional rights and responsibilities as well as mechanisms for public accountability.

"Society grants the professions authority over functions vital to itself and permits them considerable autonomy in the conduct of their affairs. In return, the professions are expected to act responsibly, always mindful of the public trust. Self-regulation to assure quality in performance is at the heart of this relationship. It is the authentic hallmark of a mature profession."[3]

People seek the services of nurses to obtain information and treatment in matters of health and illness. They use nursing care to resolve problems or manage health-promoting behaviors. Nurses help people identify both short- and long-term health goals and act as advocates for people dealing with barriers encountered in obtaining health care.[4]

Values and Assumptions

Some values and assumptions that undergird *Nursing's Social Policy Statement* are:

✦ Humans manifest an essential unity of mind/body/spirit.

✦ Human experience is contextually and culturally defined.

66

Nursing's Social Policy Statement: Second Edition

1995

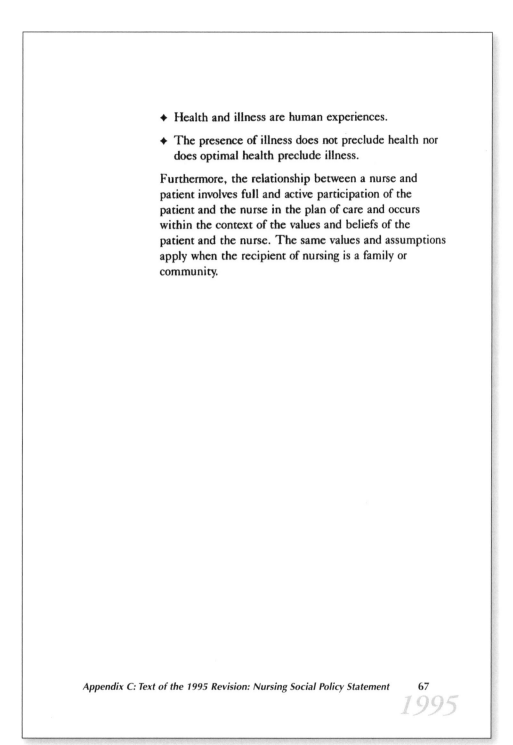

◆ Health and illness are human experiences.

◆ The presence of illness does not preclude health nor does optimal health preclude illness.

Furthermore, the relationship between a nurse and patient involves full and active participation of the patient and the nurse in the plan of care and occurs within the context of the values and beliefs of the patient and the nurse. The same values and assumptions apply when the recipient of nursing is a family or community.

Appendix C: Text of the 1995 Revision: Nursing Social Policy Statement   67

1995

DEFINITION OF NURSING

 ursing was defined in Florence Nightingale's Notes on Nursing: What It Is and What It Is Not, *published in 1859, as having "charge of the personal health of somebody . . . and what nursing has to do . . . is to put the patient in the best condition for nature to act upon him."*[5]

A century later, Virginia Henderson defined the purpose of nursing as "to assist the individual, sick or well, in the performance of those activities contributing to health or its recovery (or to a peaceful death) that he would perform unaided if he had the necessary strength, will, or

68

Nursing's Social Policy Statement: Second Edition

1995

knowledge. And to do this in such a way as to help him gain independence as rapidly as possible."[6] In the 1980 *Nursing: A Social Policy Statement*, nursing was defined as "the diagnosis and treatment of human responses to actual or potential health problems."[1]

These definitions illustrate the consistent orientation of nurses to the provision of care that promotes well-being in the people served.

These definitions illustrate the consistent orientation of nurses to the provision of care that promotes well-being in the people served. The nursing profession remains committed to the care and nurturing of both healthy and ill people, individually or in groups and communities.

Since 1980, nursing philosophy and practice have been influenced by a greater elaboration of the science of caring and its integration with the traditional knowledge base for diagnosis and treatment of human responses to health and illness. As such, definitions of nursing more frequently acknowledge four essential features of contemporary nursing practice:

◆ attention to the full range of human experiences and responses to health and illness without restriction to a problem-focused orientation;

◆ integration of objective data with knowledge gained from an understanding of the patient or group's subjective experience;

◆ application of scientific knowledge to the processes of diagnosis and treatment; and,

◆ provision of a caring relationship that facilitates health and healing.

Appendix C: Text of the 1995 Revision: Nursing Social Policy Statement　　69

1995

KNOWLEDGE BASE FOR
NURSING PRACTICE

ursing is a scientific discipline as well as a profession.

The knowledge base for nursing practice is derived from multiple sources, including nursing science, philosophy, and ethics, and physical, economic, biomedical, behavioral, and social sciences. To expand the knowledge base of the discipline, nurses generate and utilize theories and research findings that are relevant to nursing practice and fit with nursing's values about health and illness.

70

Nursing's Social Policy Statement: Second Edition

1995

Phenomena of Concern

The phenomena of concern to nurses are human experiences and responses to birth, health, illness, and death. Nurses focus on these phenomena within the context of individuals, families, groups, and communities.

Following are examples of phenomena that are foci of nursing care and research:

◆ care and self-care processes;

◆ physiological and pathophysiological processes—such as rest, sleep, respiration, circulation, reproduction, nutrition, elimination, sexuality, and communication;

◆ physical and emotional comfort, discomfort, and pain;

◆ emotions related to experiences of birth, health, illness, and death;

◆ meanings ascribed to health and illness;

◆ decision- and choice-making abilities;

◆ perceptual orientations such as self-image and control over one's body and environments;

◆ relationships, role performance, and change processes within relationships; and,

◆ social policies and their effects on the health of individuals, families, and communities.

The nurse's theoretical and research-based understandings of these phenomena and the preferences of patients, families, or communities guide the formulation of plans of care.

Appendix C: Text of the 1995 Revision: Nursing Social Policy Statement 71

1995

Interventions are recommended based on the nurse's clinical judgment about the phenomena of concern and theoretical, practical, or scientific knowledge about the relationships between potential interventions and desired outcomes.

Diagnosis

Nurses identify the human responses to actual or potential health problems they observe and name their conceptualization of the diagnosis using a variety of classification systems.[7] Diagnoses facilitate communication among health care providers and the recipients of care and provide for initial direction in choice of treatments and subsequent evaluation of the outcomes of care.

Interventions

The actions nurses take on behalf of patients, families, or communities are referred to as nursing interventions or treatments. The aim of nursing actions is to assist patients, families, and communities to improve, correct, or adjust to physical, emotional, psychosocial, spiritual, cultural, and environmental conditions for which they seek help.

Nursing interventions may be either direct or indirect. Direct care interventions are performed through interaction with patients. Indirect care interventions are performed away from the patient but on behalf of a patient or group of patients, and are aimed at management of the care environment and interdisciplinary collaboration.[8] Interventions are recommended based on the nurse's clinical judgment about the phenomena of concern and theoretical, practical, or scientific knowledge about the relationships between potential interventions and desired outcomes.

When nursing care is provided to individuals, it is provided within relationships that involve both physical and emotional intimacy. Nursing assessments, treatments, and comfort care are delivered with compassion and respect for human dignity. The interpersonal close-

72

1995

Nursing's Social Policy Statement: Second Edition

ness that develops between a nurse and patient provides a context for open discussion of the patient's experiences of health and illness. The nature of the relationship, therefore, allows the nurse to assist people effectively, whether giving physical care, providing emotional support, engaging in health teaching or counseling, or assisting recovery or a peaceful death.

Outcomes

Nursing interventions are intended to produce beneficial effects for the patient, family, or community. Nurses evaluate the effectiveness of their interventions in relation to identified outcomes and use these assessments to revise diagnoses, outcomes, and plans of care. Whenever possible, recipients of care participate in determining whether nursing actions have been effective.

Appendix C: Text of the 1995 Revision: Nursing Social Policy Statement 73

1995

SCOPE OF NURSING PRACTICE

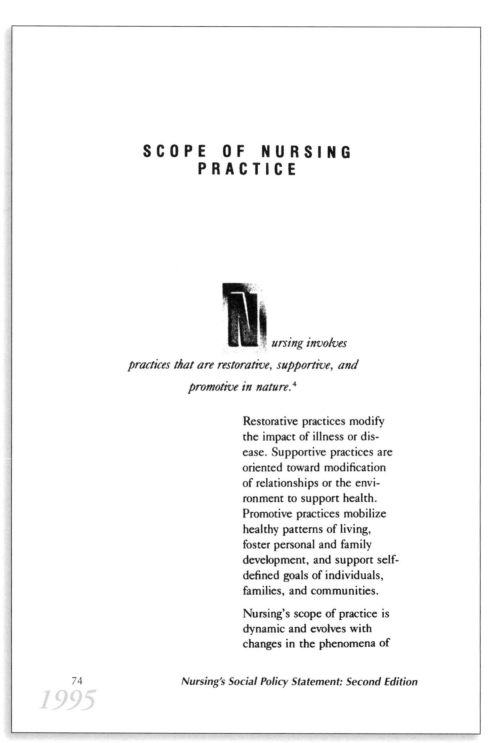

ursing involves practices that are restorative, supportive, and promotive in nature.[4]

Restorative practices modify the impact of illness or disease. Supportive practices are oriented toward modification of relationships or the environment to support health. Promotive practices mobilize healthy patterns of living, foster personal and family development, and support self-defined goals of individuals, families, and communities.

Nursing's scope of practice is dynamic and evolves with changes in the phenomena of

74

Nursing's Social Policy Statement: Second Edition

1995

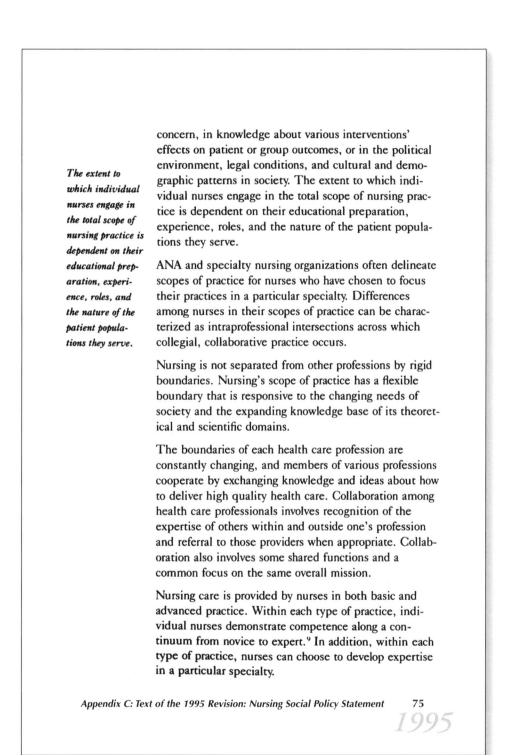

The extent to which individual nurses engage in the total scope of nursing practice is dependent on their educational preparation, experience, roles, and the nature of the patient populations they serve.

concern, in knowledge about various interventions' effects on patient or group outcomes, or in the political environment, legal conditions, and cultural and demographic patterns in society. The extent to which individual nurses engage in the total scope of nursing practice is dependent on their educational preparation, experience, roles, and the nature of the patient populations they serve.

ANA and specialty nursing organizations often delineate scopes of practice for nurses who have chosen to focus their practices in a particular specialty. Differences among nurses in their scopes of practice can be characterized as intraprofessional intersections across which collegial, collaborative practice occurs.

Nursing is not separated from other professions by rigid boundaries. Nursing's scope of practice has a flexible boundary that is responsive to the changing needs of society and the expanding knowledge base of its theoretical and scientific domains.

The boundaries of each health care profession are constantly changing, and members of various professions cooperate by exchanging knowledge and ideas about how to deliver high quality health care. Collaboration among health care professionals involves recognition of the expertise of others within and outside one's profession and referral to those providers when appropriate. Collaboration also involves some shared functions and a common focus on the same overall mission.

Nursing care is provided by nurses in both basic and advanced practice. Within each type of practice, individual nurses demonstrate competence along a continuum from novice to expert.[9] In addition, within each type of practice, nurses can choose to develop expertise in a particular specialty.

Appendix C: Text of the 1995 Revision: Nursing Social Policy Statement   75

1995

Basic Nursing Practice

Nurses who practice at the basic or entry level of practice have graduated from approved schools of nursing and have qualified by national examination for registered nurse (R.N.) licenses. Since 1965, ANA has consistently affirmed the baccalaureate degree in nursing as the preferred educational requirement for basic nursing practice.

Beyond formal education, nurses in basic practice can choose to focus their experience and continuing education on an area of specialty in nursing, and this specialized knowledge base may be acknowledged through certification. As the basis for granting certification, many credentialing bodies require the baccalaureate degree in nursing in addition to other demonstrations of knowledge in specialty practice. Although practices of individual nurses vary according to level of education, experience, competence, and role, all nurses are accountable for meeting the profession's standards of clinical practice.[10]

Nurses practicing at the basic level provide care for patients and families in environments such as homes, schools, and places of employment, as well as in hospitals, ambulatory care settings, skilled nursing facilities, long-term care institutions, protective or custodial institutions, and nurse-managed and other community-based health centers.

Based on outcomes desired, nurses intervene to promote health, prevent illness, or assist with activities that contribute to recovery from illness or to achieving a peaceful death. They may initiate treatments themselves or carry out interventions initiated by advanced practice registered nurses or other licensed health care providers.

Nurses in basic practice are coordinators of care as well as care givers. They integrate the processes of patient

76

Nursing's Social Policy Statement: Second Edition

1995

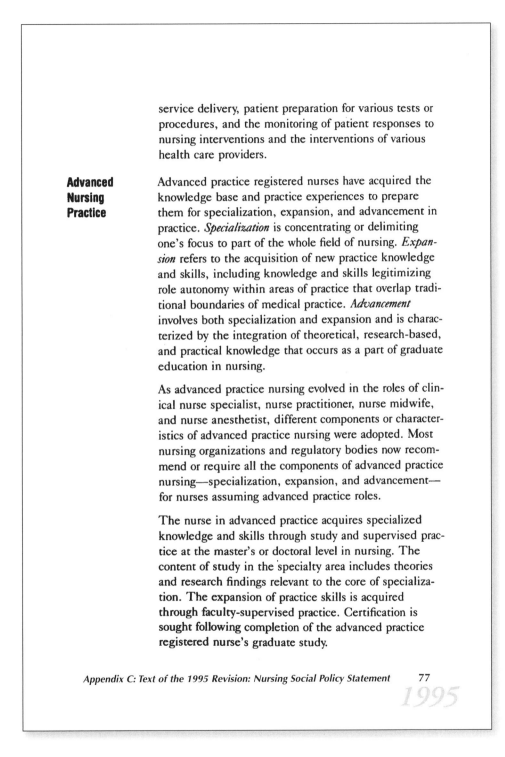

service delivery, patient preparation for various tests or procedures, and the monitoring of patient responses to nursing interventions and the interventions of various health care providers.

Advanced Nursing Practice

Advanced practice registered nurses have acquired the knowledge base and practice experiences to prepare them for specialization, expansion, and advancement in practice. *Specialization* is concentrating or delimiting one's focus to part of the whole field of nursing. *Expansion* refers to the acquisition of new practice knowledge and skills, including knowledge and skills legitimizing role autonomy within areas of practice that overlap traditional boundaries of medical practice. *Advancement* involves both specialization and expansion and is characterized by the integration of theoretical, research-based, and practical knowledge that occurs as a part of graduate education in nursing.

As advanced practice nursing evolved in the roles of clinical nurse specialist, nurse practitioner, nurse midwife, and nurse anesthetist, different components or characteristics of advanced practice nursing were adopted. Most nursing organizations and regulatory bodies now recommend or require all the components of advanced practice nursing—specialization, expansion, and advancement—for nurses assuming advanced practice roles.

The nurse in advanced practice acquires specialized knowledge and skills through study and supervised practice at the master's or doctoral level in nursing. The content of study in the specialty area includes theories and research findings relevant to the core of specialization. The expansion of practice skills is acquired through faculty-supervised practice. Certification is sought following completion of the advanced practice registered nurse's graduate study.

*Most nursing or-
ganizations and
regulatory bodies
now recommend
or require all the
components of ad-
vanced practice
nursing—speciali-
zation, expansion,
and advance-
ment—for nurses
assuming ad-
vanced practice
roles.*

The term advanced practice is used to refer exclusively to advanced *clinical* practice. Nursing practice requires that some nurses assume other advanced roles in the profession—e.g., educator, administrator, and researcher. These roles are critical to the preparation of nurses for practice, the provision of environments condu- cive to nursing practice, and the continued development of the knowledge base that nurses use in practice. Although nursing educators, administrators, and researchers are prepared educationally at the master's or doctoral level, they are not considered advanced practice registered nurses unless they possess advanced practice knowledge and skills in addition to their expertise in education, research, or administration.

Professions respond to the needs of society by identi- fying appropriate areas of specialization. As trends evolve and potential new areas of advanced practice nursing are identified, graduate programs are established by universities, the institutions with primary social responsibility for the education of scientists and profes- sionals. Among the criteria universities use to decide that a new area of practice merits establishment of a program are:

◆ The practice area lies within or would be a reasonable expansion of nursing's scope of practice.

◆ A documented need exists for health care in that area of practice.

◆ There is a body of knowledge upon which the prac- tice can be based.

◆ Faculty are available who are expert in that area by reason of clinical experience and expert knowledge.

◆ There is ample evidence that the field of nursing

78

1995

Nursing's Social Policy Statement: Second Edition

would be diminished if the recognized need were ignored.

The scope of advanced nursing practice is distinguished by autonomy to practice at the edges of the expanding boundaries of nursing's scope of practice. One hallmark of advanced practice nursing—whether in the primary care setting, the community, or the hospital—is the preponderance of self-initiated treatment regimens, as opposed to dependent functions (i.e., actions taken in response to treatments initiated by other health care providers). Because of the expanded practice and knowledge base, advanced practice nursing is also characterized by a complexity of clinical decision making and a skill in managing organizations and environments greater than that required for the practice of nursing at the basic level.

The scope of advanced nursing practice is distinguished by autonomy to practice at the edges of the expanding boundaries of nursing's scope of practice.

The advanced practice registered nurse works with individuals, families, groups, and communities to assess health needs; develop diagnoses; plan, implement and manage care; and evaluate outcomes of care. Within their specialty areas, advanced practice registered nurses may also plan and advocate care that promotes health and prevents disease and disability; direct care or manage systems of care for complex patient/family/community populations; manage acute and chronic illness, childbirth, and the care of patients before, during, and after anesthesia; and prescribe, administer, and evaluate pharmacological treatment regimens.

In addition, advanced practice registered nurses serve as mentors, consultants, and educators of nurses in basic practice. They conduct research to expand the knowledge base of nursing practice, provide leadership for practice changes, and contribute to the advancement of the profession, the health care sector, and society as a whole.

REGULATION OF NURSING PRACTICE

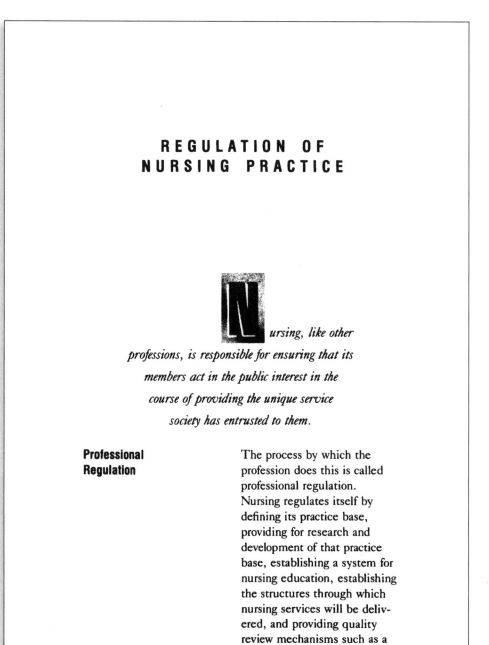

ursing, like other professions, is responsible for ensuring that its members act in the public interest in the course of providing the unique service society has entrusted to them.

Professional Regulation

The process by which the profession does this is called professional regulation. Nursing regulates itself by defining its practice base, providing for research and development of that practice base, establishing a system for nursing education, establishing the structures through which nursing services will be delivered, and providing quality review mechanisms such as a

80

Nursing's Social Policy Statement: Second Edition

1995

code of ethics, standards of practice, structures for peer review, and a system of credentialing.

Professional regulation of nursing practice begins with the profession's definition of nursing and the scope of nursing practice. Professional standards are derived from the scope of nursing practice.

ANA, in collaboration with members of its SNAs and members of other nursing organizations:

◆ establishes a code of ethics for the profession.

◆ establishes a definition of nursing.

◆ delineates the scope of nursing practice.

◆ establishes standards of clinical nursing practice.

◆ promotes the scientific foundations of nursing practice through theory development and research.

◆ specifies the appropriate academic credentials for entry into practice at basic and advanced levels, and

◆ accredits selected organizations for peer review.

The credentialing boards that are associated with ANA and specialty nursing organizations develop and implement certification examinations and procedures for nurses who want to have their specialty practice knowledge recognized by the profession. Certification is a judgment of competence made by nurses who are themselves practicing within the area of specialization. One component of the required evidence is successful completion of an examination that tests the knowledge base for the selected area of practice. Other requirements relate to the content of course work and amount of supervised practice.

Appendix C: Text of the 1995 Revision: Nursing Social Policy Statement 81

1995

Legal Regulation

All nurses are legally accountable for actions taken in the course of nursing practice as well as actions delegated by nurses to others assisting in the delivery of nursing care. Such accountability arises from the legal regulatory mechanisms of licensure and criminal and civil statutes.

All nurses are legally accountable for actions taken in the course of nursing practice as well as actions delegated by nurses to others assisting in the delivery of nursing care.

Legal contracts between society and the professions are defined by statutes and associated regulations. State nurse practice acts and related legislative and regulatory initiatives serve as the codification of nursing's obligation to act in the best interests of society. Nurse practice acts grant nurses the authority to practice and grant society the authority to sanction nurses who violate the norms of the profession and act in a manner that threatens public safety.

Society is best served when consistent definitions of the scope of nursing practice are used by states: geographic mobility of nurses is enhanced and residents of every state have access to the full range of services that nurses are able to provide. Statutory definitions of nursing should be compatible with the profession's definition of its practice base but general enough to provide for the dynamic nature of an evolving scope of nursing practice.

As advanced practice nursing has evolved, approaches to legal regulation have been based on varying interpretations of societal need and the political philosophies of state constituencies. For both professional and legal regulatory mechanisms, the goal is consistent definitions and criteria for recognition of advanced practice.

Self-Regulation

Nurses exercise autonomy and freedom within their scope of practice. This autonomy and freedom is based upon nurses' commitment to self-regulation and accountability for practice.

1995

Nursing's Social Policy Statement: Second Edition

One form of self-regulation is accountability for the knowledge base for practice. Nurses develop and maintain current knowledge and skills through formal and continuing education and, where appropriate, seek certification in their areas of practice as a method of demonstrating this accountability.

Nurses also regulate themselves as individuals through peer review of their practices. Peer review is the mechanism by which nurses are held accountable for practice based on the profession's code of ethics. Peer evaluation fosters the refinement of knowledge, skills, and clinical decision-making processes at all levels and in all areas of clinical practice.

Appendix C: Text of the 1995 Revision: Nursing Social Policy Statement   83

1995

CONCLUSION

ursing's Social Policy Statement *includes a description of nursing in the United States—the values and social responsibility of the profession, nursing's definition and scope of practice, nursing's knowledge base, and the methods by which nursing is regulated. The statement is both an accounting of nursing's professional stewardship and an expression of nursing's continuing commitment to the society it serves.*

84

1995

Nursing's Social Policy Statement: Second Edition

REFERENCES

1. American Nurses Association. 1980. *Nursing: A social policy statement.* Kansas City, MO: the Author.

2. Page, B.B. Who owns the profession? Hastings Center Report 5:5 (October 1975): 7–8.

3. Donabedian, A. 1976. Foreword in M. Phaneuf, ed. *The nursing audit: Self-Regulation in nursing practice,* 2nd ed., p. 8. New York: Appleton-Century-Crofts.

4. Pender, N. 1987. *Health promotion in nursing practice,* 2nd ed., p. 27. Norwalk, CT: Appleton & Lange.

5. Nightingale, F. 1859. *Notes on nursing: What it is and what it is not.* London: Harrison and Sons. (facsimile edition, 1946. Philadelphia: J.B. Lippincott Company).

6. Henderson, V. 1961. *Basic principles of nursing care,* p. 42. London: International Council of Nurses.

7. McCormick, K.A., Lang, N., Zielstorff, R., Milholland, K., Saba, V., Jacox, A. 1994. Toward standard classification schemes for nursing language: Recommendations of the American Nurses Association Steering Committee on Data-bases to Support Clinical Nursing Practice. *Journal of the American Medical Informatics Association* 1:421–427.

8. McCloskey, J.C., and Bulecheck, G. M., eds. 1996 (in press). *Nursing interventions classification (NIC),* 2nd ed. St. Louis: Mosby Year Book.

9. Benner, P. 1984. From novice to expert: Excellence and power in clinical nursing practice. Reading, MA: Addison-Wesley.

10. American Nurses Association. 1991. *Standards of clinical nursing practice.* Washington, DC: American Nurses Publishing.

Appendix C: Text of the 1995 Revision: Nursing Social Policy Statement   85

1995

Appendix D.

Nursing: A Social Policy Statement (1980)

The content in this appendix is not current and is of historical significance only.

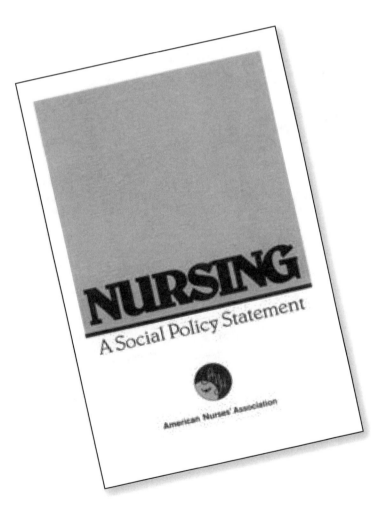

Contents

1980

Preface

During 1979 the Committee of Chairpersons of the American Nurses' Association adopted as a goal the development of a coherent policy on nursing resources and coordinated strategy for implementation of the policy, including appropriate credentialing and establishment of qualifications for entry into nursing practice. A series of program activities were proposed to achieve that goal. The chairpersons determined that the Congress for Nursing Practice should assume responsibility for defining the nature and scope of nursing practice, including a description of the characteristics of specialization in nursing. The intent of the chairpersons was that the completed document serve as the basis for ANA policy.

The Congress for Nursing Practice is the structural unit of the American Nurses' Association charged by the Bylaws with responsibility for activities dealing with the scope of nursing practice, legal aspects of nursing practice, public recognition of the significance of nursing practice to health care, and the implications for nursing practice of trends in health care.

To accomplish this work, the Congress for Nursing Practice appointed a seven-member task force. The congress acknowledges the significant contributions to the advancement of nursing practice made by the task force, and expresses its particular appreciation of the contributions to that group by Hildegard Peplau and Maria Phaneuf. Their distinguished careers have helped to shape the nursing profession, and their continuing commitment to the profession is demonstrated by their indispensable participation in the work of the task force.

The Congress for Nursing Practice is indebted to the ANA Divisions on Practice and practice councils, and to the many other nurses, both individuals and groups, who reviewed and commented on a draft of this statement circulated in June 1980. To those nurses who attended the forum on the draft held at the ANA biennial convention in Houston, Texas, in June 1980, and to those who responded verbally or in writing to the draft, the congress expresses its gratitude for the interest and insights they shared.

The congress also acknowledges its appreciation of the work of ANA staff in preparation of the statement, especially that of Katherine Goldring, editor of publications, and Ruth Lewis, director of the Nursing Practice Department.

Norma Lang, Ph.D., R.N., F.A.A.N.
Chairperson
American Nurses' Association
Congress for Nursing Practice

26 *Nursing's Social Policy Statement: Second Edition*

1980

Introduction

During the last century, the question, "What is nursing?" has been raised by nurses as well as by other health professionals, legislators, and the public. During these years, nursing has steadily responded by moving forward in its conception of its work in consonance with evolving professional and social demands. Trends well under way in nursing must now be reflected in a contemporary delineation of the nature and scope of nursing practice and a description of the characteristics of specialization in nursing.

As the professional society for nursing in the United States, the American Nurses' Association is responsible for defining and establishing the scope of nursing practice. Publication of this statement enhances ongoing professional dialogue and contributes to the work of nursing's professional society in carrying out its responsibility.

The statement includes emphasis on specialization because the development of specialization in nursing practice has been a major advance in nursing during the last three decades. The profession is therefore obliged to provide means of identifying within nursing and for the public those nurses who meet stipulated criteria as specialists, so as to assure the public that those nurses who present themselves as specialists are so qualified.

The nursing profession has reached a maturity that not only justifies but also requires a statement affirming nursing's social responsibility, made in recognition of society's right to know how that responsibility is exercised in nursing practice. The nature and scope of nursing practice and characteristics of specialization in nursing have therefore been delineated here in a social policy statement.

This statement is intended as a fundamental and undergirding delineation, providing a foundation that promotes unity in nursing in a basic and common approach to practice. The statement presents facts and values in nursing as they govern relationships to the larger professional and social context. It provides enabling definitions and descriptions, seeking to clarify the direction in which nursing has evolved and to provide a means for distinguishing between desirable and undesirable directions for future development. It is hoped that this formulation of nursing's social responsibility will further the growth of the profession and the development of nursing theory.

This delineation of the nature and scope of nursing practice is tailored to the diversity, openness, and transition characteristic of the present,

Appendix B: Text of the 1980 Original: Nursing: A Social Policy Statement   **27**

1980

actual range of nursing practice. Attempts to conceptually delimit nursing more clearly than it is actually delimited would have been potentially harmful. Such attempts would not only have been unjust to many nurses, but could be used prematurely or arbitrarily to limit the scope of nursing practice; care has been taken to avoid both of these pitfalls.

The statement is intended for use by nurses in achieving a fresh perspective on their practice, in helping the profession to move forward at a speed consistent with soundness and based on the achievements already attained, and in giving society a current view of the nature of nursing practice.

Useful as definitions and descriptions may be, they cannot accomplish what only political processes can achieve. Neither definitions nor descriptions can determine the actual scope of practice over the years ahead. Nor can they determine the relationships within nursing, between nursing and other health professions, between nursing and the various publics it serves, or between nursing and governmental bodies that formulate and direct implementation of public policy pertinent to health care systems, including the education of health professionals. It is individuals and groups working together through political processes who make these determinations. Because this social policy statement on the nature and scope of nursing practice, including its description of the characteristics of specialization in nursing, attests to nursing's social responsibilities, use of it by the individuals and groups who make the determinations that influence current developments and the shape of the future is essential.

The 1980s have been identified as a decade of decision in nursing. The social policy statement has been so cast as to facilitate decisions through which nursing can consolidate achievements of the past and move with wisdom and courage into its future of service to society.

28   *Nursing's Social Policy Statement: Second Edition*

1980

I. The Social Context of Nursing

Nursing, like other professions, is an essential part of the society out of which it grew and with which it has been evolving. Nursing can be said to be owned by society, in the sense that nursing's professional interest must be and must be perceived as serving the interests of the larger whole of which it is a part. The mutually beneficial relationship between society and its profession has been expressed as follows:

> A profession acquires recognition, relevance, and even meaning in terms of its relationship to that society, its culture and institutions, and its other members. Professions acquire recognition and relevance primarily in terms of needs, conditions, and traditions of particular societies and their members. It is societies (and often vested interests within them) that determine, in accord with their different technological and economic levels of development and their socioeconomic, political and cultural conditions, and values, what professional skills and knowledge they most need and desire. By various financial means, institutions will then emerge to train interested individuals to supply those needs.

> Logically, then, the professions open to individuals in any particular society are the property not of the individual but of society. What individuals acquire through training is professional knowledge and skill, not a profession or even part ownership of one.[1]

Some Current Social Concerns and Directions in Health Care

Health care is currently a major focus of attention in the United States. Public and political determinations are being made in five major areas, in each of which nursing has leadership responsibilities:

1. Organization, delivery, and financing of health care. Attention to this area has been sharpened by the costs of care, which threaten to rise beyond the finite national economic capabilities, and by a public morality that requires a general availability, accessibility, and acceptability of health care.

2. Continuing development of health resources, including facilities and manpower for personal care and community health services, in a manner consistent with available knowledge and technology, and an increasing focus on individuals, families, and other groups as basic self-help resources.

Appendix B: Text of the 1980 Original: Nursing: A Social Policy Statement   29

1980

3. Provision for the public health through use of preventive and environmental measures, and increased assumption of responsibility by individuals, families, and other groups as basic self-help resources.

4. Development of new knowledge and technology through research.

5. Health care planning as a matter of national policy and related regulations, made specific by the National Health Planning and Resources Development Act of 1974 (Public Law 93-641).

In these and other areas, public determinations find expression through political processes carried out by governmental and voluntary bodies. The political process includes the identification of public needs and demands and of the resources available to meet them, combined with appropriation and allocation of funds to support the resources. The political process also can be and is used to shape public perceptions of needs, and thus to create public demands. At best, such use of the political process is made out of impartial concerns for the public good. At worst, it occurs for the advancement of vested interests, with the public good being of lesser or no concern. For nursing, the public good must be the overriding concern.

Through political channels in our democracy, public determinations in the five areas previously mentioned are being made in a time of transition from a disease-oriented to a health-oriented system of health care. The transition is occurring in part because of the rising costs of hospital and related medical care. When the costs of the care of the sick rise so strikingly, questions are raised about the possibility of reducing costs by preventing or controlling disease or illness by focusing on attaining, maintaining, and regaining health.

Transition from a disease-oriented to a health-oriented system of care is an evolutionary process; such processes occur over time, at a slow pace, and they are often characterized by some denial that change is occurring or that it is even possible. Health care planning as a matter of national policy is evidence that change to a health-oriented system has at least been initiated. This new focus is symbolized by the use of the words *health care* in place of *medical care* and by the increasing use of the term *health center* for hospital. The newly perceived importance of ambulatory care, primary care, and family care centers, home health services, and other patterns of care, the increasing utilization of such types of care, and the provision of public and private payment for it clearly show the impact of the evolving health orientation.

30   *Nursing's Social Policy Statement: Second Edition*

1980

While the health orientation can help to prevent, modify, or limit disease or illness, it cannot eliminate them. This change in approach in no way detracts from professional or institutional responsibility for care of the sick. In the movement to a health-oriented system of care, care of the sick remains a basic responsibility.

What is equally important is the growing realization that individuals, families, and groups have considerable responsibility for their personal health and for development of their potentials for achieving it. A public increasingly knowledgeable about health and health care systems is becoming more and more involved in related public and political decisions.

The decisions to come will be influenced by experience during the past two decades. The decade of the 1960s was characterized by the national spending of health care dollars without interfering in any way with the existing structure of the health care system. The decade of the 1970s was an era of new regulations designed to control the financial obligations resulting from the spending in the sixties. Regulation in its various forms was expensive, poorly designed, and largely ineffective.[2]

It is logical to anticipate that the 1980s will be a decade of increasing regulations with regard to the quantity, costs, and quality of health care. Because these elements are inextricably interwoven, increased attention will be concentrated on social and political options in health care. The development of social and political priorities for action will depend on choice among options, based on society's values and its needs.

Selected Specific Areas of Concern to Nursing

Nursing helps to serve society's interests in the area of health. The nursing profession has made and continues to make a substantial contribution toward evolution of a health-oriented system of care. Nursing practice has been health-oriented for more than half a century, partly because of its focus on individuals as persons and on the family as the necessary unit of service. In nursing so practiced, the current health movement was foreshadowed.

Health is a dynamic state of being in which the developmental and behavioral potential of an individual is realized to the fullest extent possible. Each human being possesses various strengths and limitations resulting from the interaction of environmental and hereditary factors. The relative dominance of the strengths and limitations determines an individual's place on the health continuum; it determines the person's biological and behavioral integrity, his wholeness.[3]

Appendix B: Text of the 1980 Original: Nursing: A Social Policy Statement   31

1980

During periods of illness, trauma, or disability, an individual or family may require varying degrees of personal assistance in coping with a manifest problem, with the treatment plan designed to alleviate the problem, or with the sequelae. An individual or family may require varying degrees of assistance to obtain information in matters of health, to receive anticipatory guidance and therapeutic counseling to resolve problems, or to manage usual health practices, both during periods of wellness and when faced with a progressive or long-term health problem.

Viewed in this light, health becomes the center of nursing attention, not as an end in itself, but as a means to life that is meaningful and manageable.[4] Professional practice entails recognition that:

> Man has an inherent capacity for change in constructive and destructive directions. Access to opportunities for growth and possible change is every person's right, regardless of social or economic status, personal attributes, or the nature of the health problems. . . . Individual differences influence not only a person's potential for change, but also the meanings and values associated with it. Helping services that are founded on respect for human dignity recognize possibilities for individual freedom of choice and enhance opportunities for conscious self direction.[5]

A Nursing View of Working Relationships in Health Care

The nursing profession is particularly concerned with the working relationships essential to the carrying out of its health-oriented mission. The complexity and size of the health care system and its transitional state, increasing public involvement in health policy and a national focus on health, and the professionalization of nursing—all of these factors combine to intensify the importance of the direct human interactions inherent in nursing's response to human needs and society's expectations.

Nursing involvement in these interactions needs to be carried on with explicit assessment of the nature of working relationships. Conceptually there are three basic types of working relationships.[6] The first and most primitive is the one in which one person commands another. The second type can be identified as detente. The third level is collaboration.

In the first type, the person with power gives the command, which another obeys. In so commanding, the assumption is usually made that little knowledge, few skills, and little or no judgment or initiative are entailed in responding to the command. In health care, that assumption is generally false; the human beings involved have the

32

Nursing's Social Policy Statement: Second Edition

1980

capacity to exercise judgment, as warranted by the relevant knowledge and skills. This first level is essentially the master-slave relationship.

Detente implies power on both sides that is recognized by both, a recognition and acceptance of separate spheres of activity and responsibility, reciprocal acceptance of the legitimate interests of both parties, and some mutuality of interests and commonality of goals that are recognized by both parties. Detente may be likened to armed neutrality. It is a little-acknowledged prerequisite to genuine collaboration.

Collaboration means true partnership, in which the power on both sides is valued by both, with recognition and acceptance of separate and combined spheres of activity and responsibility, mutual safeguarding of the legitimate interests of each party, and a commonality of goals that is recognized by both parties. This is a relationship based upon recognition that each is richer and more truly real because of the strength and uniqueness of the other.

In practice, working relationships are rarely pure in type, even within individuals. Working relationships generally combine characteristics of the three types and vary with specific circumstances. In groups and in society as a whole there has been movement away from the command-obey type of relationship, through the detente type of interaction, toward collaboration, due to changes of a social and political nature affecting each of the health professions and the health care system. This change is part of the process of democratization that has been occurring for hundreds of years and has accelerated in the twentieth century.

Nursing must recognize and assess the nature of working relationships with patients and families, and with other health professionals and health workers, as well as relationships within nursing and between nursing and representatives of the public at large.

Authority for Nursing Practice

The authority for nursing, as for other professions, is based on a social contract, which in turn derives from a complex social base.

> There is a social contract between society and the professions. Under its terms, society grants the professions authority over functions vital to itself and permits them considerable autonomy in the conduct of their own affairs. In return, the professions are expected to act responsibly, always mindful of the public trust. Self-regulation to assure quality in performance is at the heart of this relationship. It is the authentic hallmark of a mature profession.[7]

Appendix B: Text of the 1980 Original: Nursing: A Social Policy Statement   33

1980

As is necessary to a profession, nursing has a professional society—the American Nurses' Association — through which its responsibility to a society as a whole is exercised. Nursing's professional society performs an essential function in articulating and strengthening, as well as maintaining, the social contract that exists between nursing and society, upon which the authority to practice nursing is based.

That social contract has been made specific through the professional society's work derived from the collective expertise of its members, such as (1) establishing a code of ethics[8]; (2) establishing standards of practice[9]; (3) fostering development of nursing theory, derived from nursing research into those conditions that are the focus of practice, so as to explain observations and guide nursing actions; (4) establishing educational requirements for entry into professional practice[10]; (5) developing certification processes for the profession; and (6) other developmental work directed toward making more specific nursing's accountability to society.

One of the consequences of these and other of nursing's self-regulatory activities has been enactment of nursing practice acts and related licensure legislation and regulations that make specific the legal authority to practice. This legal authority to practice stems from the social contract between society and the profession; the social contract does not derive from legislation.

34

Nursing's Social Policy Statement: Second Edition

1980

II. The Nature and Scope of Nursing Practice

A Definition of Nursing

In Nightingale's *Notes on Nursing: What It Is and What It Is Not,* published in 1859, nursing is defined as to have "charge of the personal health of somebody . . . and what nursing has to do . . . is to put the patient in the best condition for nature to act upon him."[11] A century later, Henderson defined nursing as "to assist the individual, sick or well, in the performance of those activities contributing to health or its recovery (or to a peaceful death) that he would perform unaided if he had the necessary strength, will or knowledge. And to do this in such a way as to help him gain independence as rapidly as possible."[12]

These definitions illustrate the consistent orientation of nurses to the provision of care that promotes well being in the people served. The nursing profession remains committed to the care and nurturing of sick and well people, individually and in groups.

The definition of nursing presented here maintains this historical orientation and at the same time reflects the influence of nursing theory that is a part of nursing's evolution:

> *Nursing is the diagnosis and treatment of human responses to actual or potential health problems.*

This definition is based on language proposed in 1970 by the New York State Nurses Association.[13] This language was adopted as part of the Nurse Practice Act of New York State in 1972 and later incorporated in the nursing practice acts of several other states.[14, 15]

This definition points to four defining characteristics of nursing: phenomena, theory application, nursing action, and evaluation of effects of action in relation to phenomena.

Phenomena: The phenomena of concern to nurses are human responses to actual or potential health problems. Any observable manifestation, need, condition, concern, event, dilemma, difficulty, occurrence, or fact that can be described or scientifically explained and is within the target area of nursing practice is of interest to nurses. The human responses of people toward which the actions of nurses are directed are of two kinds: (1) reactions of individuals and groups to actual health problems (health-restoring responses), such as the impact of illness effects upon the self and family, and related self-care needs; and (2) concerns of individuals and groups about potential health

Appendix B: Text of the 1980 Original: Nursing: A Social Policy Statement 35

1980

problems (health-supporting responses), such as monitoring and teaching in populations or communities at risk in which educative needs for information, skill development, health-oriented attitudes, and related behavioral changes arise.

Nursing addresses itself to a wide range of health-related responses observed in sick and well persons. Those responses can be reactions to an actual problem, such as a disease, or they can anticipate a potential health problem. The difference between the response to a health problem and the problem itself is worth noting, as it is here where an intermeshing and complementarity of the distinct foci of the practices of nursing and medicine occur. Human responses to health problems, the phenomena to which the actions of nurses are directed, are often multiple, episodic, or continuous, fluid, and varying, and are less discrete or circumscribed than medical diagnostic categories tend to be.

The following provides an illustrative list rather than a comprehensive taxonomy of the human responses that are the focus for nursing intervention:

1. Self-care limitations

2. Impaired functioning in areas such as rest, sleep, ventilation, circulation, activity, nutrition, elimination, skin, sexuality, and the like

3. Pain and discomfort

4. Emotional problems related to illness and treatment, life-threatening events, or daily life experiences, such as anxiety, loss, loneliness, and grief

5. Distortion of symbolic functions, reflected in interpersonal and intellectual processes, such as hallucinations

6. Deficiencies in decision making and ability to make personal choices

7. Self-image changes required by health status

8. Dysfunctional perceptual orientations to health

9. Strains related to life processes, such as birth, growth and development, and death

10. Problematic affiliative relationships.

36   *Nursing's Social Policy Statement: Second Edition*

1980

The nature of phenomena to which the actions of nurses are directed is ascertained by assessment in its various forms, such as observation, interviewing, measurement, and the like. Instruments for the measurement of conditions within the purview of nursing are being developed and tested through nursing research.[16]

Diagnosis is a beginning effort to objectify a perceived difficulty or need by naming it, as a basis for understanding and taking action to resolve the concern. A nurse's conceptualization or diagnosis of a presenting condition is a way of ascribing meaning to it, which may or may not accurately reflect the phenomenon under consideration for treatment. Both the diagnosis and its theoretical interpretation are open to revision; indeed, in some modalities, such as psychotherapy, diagnostic revision is simultaneous with the ongoing therapeutic work.

Theory: Nurses use theory in the form of concepts, principles, processes, and the like, to sharpen their observations and to understand the phenomena within the domain of nursing practice. Such understanding precedes and serves as a basis for determining nursing actions to be taken.

The theoretical base for nursing is partially self-generated and partially drawn from other fields; the resulting insights are integrated into a foundation for nursing practice. Nursing is primarily an applied science: it uses the results of nursing research (which tend to be specifically related to the human responses of concern to nurses) and it selects theories from many other sciences on the basis of their explanatory value in relation to the phenomena nurses diagnose and treat.

The range of theories nurses use includes intrapersonal, interpersonal, and systems theories. Intrapersonal theories explain within-person phenomena. Interpersonal theories aid understanding of interactions between two or more people. Systems theories provide explanations of complex networks or organizations, the dynamics of their parts and processes in interaction. Use of this range of theories is necessary because the various conditions within the purview of nursing cannot be understood in terms of cause-effect relations only, but also require knowledge of system dynamics, pattern and process interactions.

When responses to actual health problems are being treated, the nature of the difficulty and its causes (when known) require theory application for full understanding of extant problems. When responses to potential health problems or maintenance of health are the focus for the nursing action, theories that aid conceptualization of optimal

Appendix B: Text of the 1980 Original: Nursing: A Social Policy Statement 37

1980

functioning of individual capacities and processes and of the dynamics of human systems are applied to determine reordering of behavior or life styles congruent with healthy living. Thus, theory selected for application in nursing practice is chosen for its relevance to the task at hand.

The ideas and theories of the individual practitioner influence nursing practice in focus and action. Ideally, the actions of the nurse are taken from a theoretical base that includes an accurate understanding of the phenomena in question and a means for evaluation or readjustment.

Actions: The aims of nursing actions are to ameliorate, improve, or correct conditions to which those practices are directed, to prevent illness, and to promote health. Ideally, actions are taken on the basis of understood fact (phenomena). In carrying out nursing care, highly developed technical and interpersonal skills are equally as important as the sensitive observation and intellectual competencies required for the nurse in the nursing situation to arrive at a diagnosis (explanation of a problem at hand) and determination of beneficial nursing actions to be taken. Treatment of a diagnosed condition involves nursing actions that can be described and explained theoretically as to their relation to phenomena and expected outcome

Effects: Nursing actions are intended to produce beneficial effects in relation to identified responses. It is the results of the evaluation of outcomes of nursing actions that suggest whether or not those actions have been effective in improving or resolving the conditions to which they were directed. The results of research study of the relation of particular actions to specific phenomena, determined under controlled conditions, provide more rigorous scientific evidence of beneficial effects to nursing actions than does periodic evaluation or testimonials as to effectiveness.

Nursing values an approach to practice in which investigation and action are interrelated. This approach is apparent in the four characteristics of nursing, which have been described, and is reflected in the use of the nursing process, which serves as an organizing framework for practice.

The nursing process encompasses all significant steps taken in the care of the patients, with attention to their rationale, their sequence, and relative importance in helping the patient reach specified and attainable health goals. The nursing process requires a systematic approach to the assessment of the patient's situation, which includes reconciliation of patient/family and nurse perceptions of the situation; a plan for nursing actions, which includes

38   *Nursing's Social Policy Statement: Second Edition*

1980

patient/family participation in goal setting; joint implementation of the plan; and evaluation which includes patient/family participation. The steps in the process are not necessarily taken in strict sequence beginning with assessment and ending with evaluation. The steps may be taken concurrently and should be taken recurrently, as in the evaluation of the assessment or the plan of action.[17]

Recognition of the nursing process is reflected in the ANA Standards of Nursing Practice, which apply to all nursing practice. These standards, published by the professional society in 1973, provide one broad basis for evaluation of practice and reflect recognition of the rights of the person receiving nursing care. The standards describe a "therapeutic alliance" of the nurse and the person for whom she or he provides care through use of the nursing process.[18]

The relationship between the characteristics of nursing, the nursing process, and the standards that reflect it are shown in Figure 1. The characteristics of phenomena and theory application are implicit in the standards involving data collection, diagnosis, and planning; that of action is referenced in the standards involving planning and treatment; and the characteristic of effects is related to the standards involving evaluation and revision.

Scope of Nursing Practice

Nursing is a segment of the health care system. In addition to the care an individual provides for his own health, health care is provided through the services of many professions, including nursing, medicine, pharmacy, social work, and dentistry, among others. The term *health care* is therefore not synonymous with nursing care or medical care, but refers to a composite of planned care provided by interdependent professions whose members collaborate with individuals and groups being served. Health care includes many professional segments, each of which has its own definite characteristics and independent functions.

As is true for any profession, the continuity, growth, and thriving of nursing are contingent upon education, research, and administration. Other statements of the American Nurses' Association describe these components of the nursing profession.[19,20,21]

The scope of nursing practice, the contents of the nursing segment of health care, has four defining characteristics: boundary, intersections, dimensions, and core.

Appendix B: Text of the 1980 Original: Nursing: A Social Policy Statement   39

1980

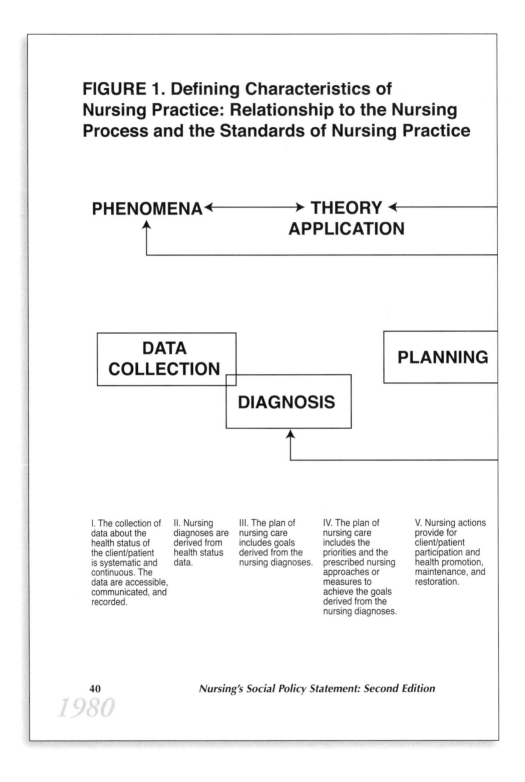

FIGURE 1. Defining Characteristics of Nursing Practice: Relationship to the Nursing Process and the Standards of Nursing Practice

PHENOMENA ←→ THEORY ←
                 APPLICATION

DATA COLLECTION

DIAGNOSIS

PLANNING

I. The collection of data about the health status of the client/patient is systematic and continuous. The data are accessible, communicated, and recorded.

II. Nursing diagnoses are derived from health status data.

III. The plan of nursing care includes goals derived from the nursing diagnoses.

IV. The plan of nursing care includes the priorities and the prescribed nursing approaches or measures to achieve the goals derived from the nursing diagnoses.

V. Nursing actions provide for client/patient participation and health promotion, maintenance, and restoration.

40   *Nursing's Social Policy Statement: Second Edition*

1980

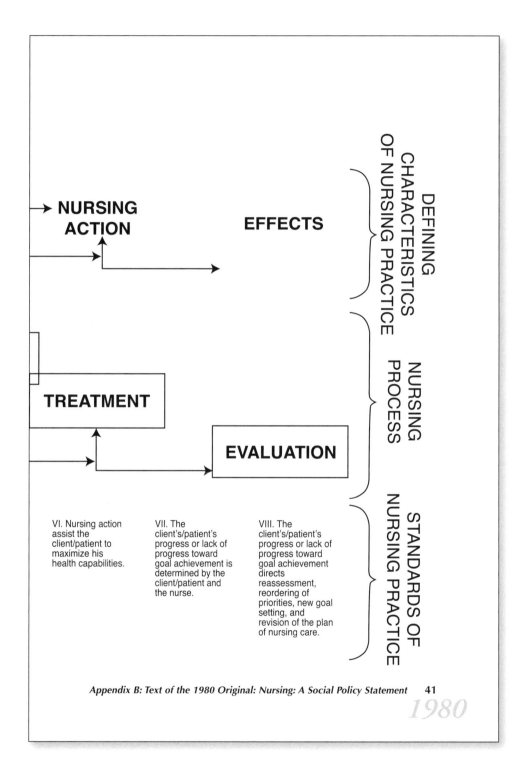

NURSING
ACTION

EFFECTS

DEFINING
CHARACTERISTICS
OF NURSING PRACTICE

TREATMENT

EVALUATION

NURSING PROCESS

STANDARDS OF
NURSING PRACTICE

VI. Nursing action
assist the
client/patient to
maximize his
health capabilities.

VII. The
client's/patient's
progress or lack of
progress toward
goal achievement is
determined by the
client/patient and
the nurse.

VIII. The
client's/patient's
progress or lack of
progress toward
goal achievement
directs
reassessment,
reordering of
priorities, new goal
setting, and
revision of the plan
of nursing care.

Appendix B: Text of the 1980 Original: Nursing: A Social Policy Statement   **41**

1980

Boundary: The nursing segment of health care has an external boundary that expands outward in response to changing needs, demands, and capacities of society. As is true of all professions, nursing is dynamic rather than static. As new needs and demands impinge upon nursing, and as a consequence of nursing research, the other three defining characteristics of scope begin to change, resulting in expansion of the boundary.

Intersections: The nursing segment of health care intersects with other professions involved in health care. These interprofessional interfacings are meeting points at which nursing extends its practice into the domains of other professions. These intersections are not hard and fast lines separating nursing from another profession; the relations between nursing and medicine at these interfacings are especially fluid and unproblematic in situations in which collegial, collaborative joint practice obtains.[22] All of the health care professions interact, share the same overall mission, have access to the same published scientific knowledge, and in some degree overlap in their activities.

A statement of the scope of nursing ought not to limit the boundary or fix the intersections of nursing with other professions, but should allow for expansion and flexibility. Individual nurses, however, do limit the scope of their practice in light of their education, knowledge, competence, and interest. These differences constitute intraprofessional intersections. All nurses locate themselves somewhere within the scope of nursing on the basis of preparation for the work. Tolerance of differences in interests, in part or whole, and intraprofessional collaboration among nurses serve their shared mission: to promote health.

Core: The core of nursing practice is the basis for nursing care—the phenomena previously described. These conditions are brought into focus by naming or diagnosing them, or by hypothesizing or inferring when the facts are unclear or no diagnosis exists. Diagnosis of phenomena leads to application of theory to explain the condition and to determine actions to be taken—otherwise, diagnosis is mere labeling.

The range of diagnostic categories within the scope of nursing practice is constantly undergoing expansion. The American Nurses' Association, through its five Divisions on Nursing Practice, has identified and is further formulating the phenomena of concern that lie within the scope of responsibility of professional nurses. Various individuals and groups are presently developing classification systems of nursing diagnoses.[23,24,25]

Dimensions: The dimensions of nursing practice are characteristics that fall within and further describe the scope of nursing. A compre-

42   *Nursing's Social Policy Statement: Second Edition*

1980

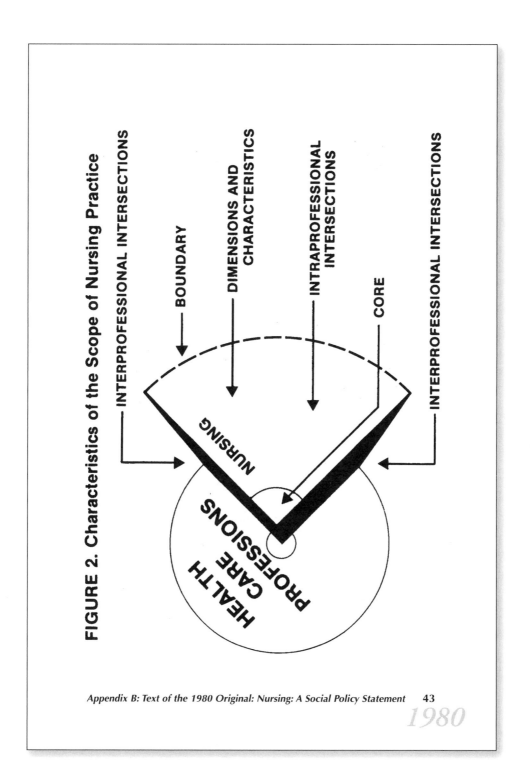

FIGURE 2. Characteristics of the Scope of Nursing Practice

Appendix B: Text of the 1980 Original: Nursing: A Social Policy Statement   43

1980

hensive statement of these characteristics would include but not be limited to descriptions of what philosophy and ethics guide nurses; what responsibilities, functions, roles, and skills characterize their work; what scientific theories they use and by what methods they apply them; where and when they practice; and with what legal authority nurses function.

One of the most distinguishing characteristics of nursing is that it involves practices that are nurturant, generative, or protective in nature.[26] They are developed to meet the health needs of individuals as integrated persons rather than as biological systems. The nurturant or nurturing behaviors provide comfort and therapy in the presence of illness or disease and foster personal development. The generative behaviors are oriented to development of new behaviors and modification of environments or systems to promote health-conducive adaptive responses of the individuals to health care crises or problems. The protective behaviors involve surveillance, assessment, and intervention in support of adaptive capabilities and developmental functions of persons. These nurse behaviors are responsive to people with conditions diagnosed and treated by nurses as they apply theory in order to explain and to guide nurse action in practice.

Nurses are guided by a humanistic philosophy having caring coupled with understanding and purpose as its central feature. Nurses have the highest regard for self-determination, independence, and choice in decision making in matters of health. Recognizing that illness and physical handicap tend to erode these attributes of persons, nursing throughout its history has provided health teaching, sharing its expertise with the public through, for example, courses in home health nursing. Presently, nursing is directing its attention to evolving theory and practices focusing on the responsibility of the individual for his own health.

Nurses are committed to respecting human beings because of a profound regard for humanity. This principle applies to themselves, to people receiving care, and to other people who share in the provision of care, as well as to humanity in general. This basic commitment is unaltered by the social, educational, economic, cultural, racial, religious, or other specific attributes of the human beings receiving care, including the nature and duration of disease and illness.

Nursing care is provided in an interpersonal relationship process of nurse-with-a-patient, nurse-with-a-family, nurse-with-a-group. It involves privileged intimacy—physical and interpersonal. Nursing is a laying-on-of-hands practice in which nurses have access to the body of another person in carrying out assessments, comfort care, and defini-

44   *Nursing's Social Policy Statement: Second Edition*

1980

tive treatments. At best, nurses carry out such physical ministrations with compassion and with recognition of the client's dignity. Nursing is a practice in which interpersonal closeness of a professional kind develops and aids the investigation and discussion of problems, as nurse and patient (or family or group) seek jointly to resolve those concerns. Nursing therefore includes an array of functions, including physical care, anticipatory guidance, health teaching, counseling, and the like.

Nursing practice demands professional intention and commitment carried out in accordance with the American Nurses' Association Standards of Nursing Practice and its ethical code. While all nurses are responsible for practicing in accordance with the ANA Standards of Nursing Practice, the level and sophistication of application vary with the education and skills of the individual nurse. Nursing is practiced by nurses who are generalists and by nurses who are specialists. Each nurse remains accountable for the quality of her or his practice within the full scope of nursing practice.

Generalists in nursing provide most of the care for most of the people served by nursing. In other words, in numbers and in amount of service provided, generalists provide the bulk of nursing care. The care provided by these nurses should be available to people wherever they may be at a given point in time and whatever may be their situation in terms of health, disease, illness, or injury at the time. The nurse generalist has a comprehensive approach to health care and can meet diversified health concerns of individuals, families, and communities.

Specialists in nursing are experts in providing care focused on specific clusters of phenomena drawn from the range of general practice. Specialization involves adding to the generic base of nursing practice an organized and systematized body of knowledge and competencies within a discrete area of nursing, applied through specialized practice. Specialized nursing practice represents a refining of interests, either by focusing upon a part of the whole of nursing practice or by focusing upon relations among parts. The phenomena of concerns selected by specialists in nursing practice may relate either to a specialized field or to the interrelation among specialized fields.

All nurses practicing with patients and with persons seeking health address the phenomena that form the core of nursing practice. Variations within nursing practice resulting from differences in level of education, extent of experience, and competence occur in regard to the following:

- Assessment and data collection

Appendix B: Text of the 1980 Original: Nursing: A Social Policy Statement   **45**

1980

- Analysis of data

- Application of theory

- Breadth and depth of knowledge base, especially clinical, psychosocial, and patho/physiological theories relating to nursing diagnosis and treatment

- The range of nursing techniques

- Need for, kind, and extent of supervision by other nurses in practice

- Evaluation of effects of practice

- Identification of relationships among phenomena, nursing actions, and effects (outcomes for the patients).

All nurses are responsible for the inclusion of preventive nursing as part of general and specialized practice. Prevention in nursing is directed to promotion of health and disease prevention; securing prompt attention for medical diagnosis and treatment of disease, or as necessary when predisposition to a given disease is apparent from the nursing diagnosis; and early recognition and management of complications and other consequences due to disease or therapy.

Nurses provide care to people in various states of their life span, from birth. through death. Service is provided in environments such as homes, schools, and places of employment, as well as in general and specialty hospitals, ambulatory care settings, skilled nursing facilities, long-term care institutions, protective or custodial institutions, and in newer types of health care settings that are evolving.

All nurses are ethically and legally accountable for actions taken in the course of nursing practice as well as for actions delegated by the nurse to others assisting in the delivery of nursing care. Such accountability may be accomplished through the regulatory mechanism of licensure, through criminal and civil laws, through the code of ethics of the profession, and through peer evaluation.

46

Nursing's Social Policy Statement: Second Edition

1980

III. Specialization in Nursing Practice

Specialization is a mark of the advancement of the nursing profession. It suggests that nursing has moved from a global to a more specific way of looking at the field and its practices. Instead of homogeneity (a nurse is a nurse is a nurse), there is a heterogeneity of clinical interests and levels of competence within nursing. Such differentiation, which is a criterion of development, is occurring due to the greater complexity within the whole of nursing practice at this juncture in nursing's history.

Specialization means a narrowed focus on a part of the whole field of nursing. It entails application of a broad range of theories to selected phenomena within the domain of nursing, in order to secure depth of understanding as a basis for advances in nursing practice. It requires identification and more concentrated effort toward resolution of heretofore poorly understood questions related to the phenomena of concern to nurses. It involves empirical and controlled research to clarify aspects of a delimited part of the field of nursing, and to generate refinement of existing nursing practices, or to evolve new ones more likely to be more beneficial to clients or patients.

Specialization arises in five main ways:

- The amount and complexity of knowledge and technology create a demand for a few professionals to give special attention to applications in delimited practice areas.

- A few professional pioneers seek to obtain greater depth of understanding of phenomena related to a segment of nursing and to test new practices intended to correct or ameliorate recognized conditions.

- Public attention and available funds become focused on an area of practice in which heretofore there has been a lack of interest, knowledge, and skilled practitioners.

- The complexity of services exceeds the prevailing knowledge and skills of general practitioners, and this problem is approached by intense personal studies or post-basic study by a few interested professionals.

- Part of a professional field expands, and simultaneously some of its members seek ways for expanded use of their intellectual and other capacities.

Appendix B: Text of the 1980 Original: Nursing: A Social Policy Statement   47

1980

Specialization in nursing has been discussed since the turn of the century.[27] Initially, the term *specialist* designated nurses who had graduated from specialized hospitals, or private-duty nurses who worked only with particular kinds of patients. As early as 1910, in ANA convention proceedings, nurses were referred to as specialists. These designations, however, were based upon practical experience or indicated completion of hospital-based "post-graduate" courses in the area of nursing. These courses, which used nurses to provide nursing care but offered little by way of education as it is now known, became so numerous by the early 1940s that the National League for Nursing Education established a committee to study this matter. The committee produced guidelines for advanced courses in nursing.[28]

During the same period, advanced clinical courses began to be offered by various colleges and universities, with the assistance of government funds. The number of nurses holding baccalaureates was exceedingly small at the time, and the university-based advanced courses led to either a bachelor's or a master's degree.

In the 1950s, the meaning of the term *advanced clinical nurse* began to change as universities offered programs for preparation as "clinical specialists in nursing."[29] It was not until the 1960s, however, that all post-basic education for specialization in clinical nursing was provided in graduate programs. By 1980, over 75 colleges and universities offered such programs.[30]

Specialization in nursing is now clearly established. The process has brought about reexamination and revitalization of the generic foundation in which the specialization is rooted. Requirement of the baccalaureate for entry into professional practice, of advanced learning for specialty practice, administration, and teaching, and of doctoral education that includes focus on research capabilities emerges as necessary to fulfillment of nursing's social responsibility.

Specialization in nursing practice assists in clarifying, revising, and strengthening existing practice. It also permits new applications of knowledge and refined nursing practices to flow from the specialist to the generalist in nursing practice and graduate to basic nursing education, thus ensuring progress in the general practice of nursing.

It provides career options, including private practice, for nurses who have particular interests in a part of the nursing field and who seek greater development and use of their abilities as well as increased responsibility and authority in practice. Specialization expedites production of new knowledge and its application in practice. Specialization also provides preparation for teaching and research related to a defined area of nursing.

48   *Nursing's Social Policy Statement: Second Edition*

1980

Criteria for Specialists in Nursing Practice

The specialist in nursing practice is a nurse who, through study and supervised practice at the graduate level (master's or doctorate), has become expert in a defined area of knowledge and practice in a selected clinical area of nursing. Specialists in nursing practice are also generalists, in that they hold a baccalaureate in nursing, and therefore are able to provide the full range of nursing care. In addition, upon completion of a graduate degree in a university graduate program with an emphasis on clinical specialization, the specialist in nursing practice should meet the criteria for specialty certification through nursing's professional society.

Graduate study for preparation as a specialist in nursing practice includes in-depth study of theories relevant to the particular area of specialization and faculty-supervised clinical practice. Faculty supervision means substantial review of data obtained by the graduate student during clinical practice with clients, families, groups, or communities, whichever is required by the focus of the nurse's intended specialization. Such supervisory review is provided on a regularly scheduled basis, over a period of time of sufficient length to provide an in-depth picture of the student's developing competence as a clinical specialist.

Those competencies include ability to observe, conceptualize, diagnose, and analyze complex clinical or non-clinical problems related to health, ability to consider a wide range of theory relevant to understanding those problems, and ability to select and justify application of theory deemed to be most useful in understanding the problems and in determining the range of possible treatment options. Ability to foresee and discuss short- and long-range possible consequences is also to be demonstrated. While this is not an exhaustive list, the foregoing intellectual competencies are of the utmost importance in specialization.

The faculty member who supervises nurses who are preparing for clinical specialization functions as a role model, demonstrating intense interest in the problems germane to the specialty area and expertise regarding the knowledge and practice of that area. Faculty supervisors are also "gatekeepers," permitting only those nurses who achieve a higher level of competence for specialty practice to obtain the graduate degree and recommendation for certification as a specialist. All universities that offer graduate programs in nursing practice should be knowledgeable about requirements for certification of specialists and should inform prospective students whether or not the graduate study to be undertaken is congruent with such requirements.

Appendix B: Text of the 1980 Original: Nursing: A Social Policy Statement   **49**

1980

Certification of specialists in nursing practice is a judgment made by the profession, upon review of an array of evidence examined by a selected panel of nurses who are themselves specialists and who represent the area of specialization.

Specialists in nursing practice thus must meet two primary criteria*: (1) an earned graduate degree (master's degree or doctorate) that represents study of scientific knowledge and supervised advanced clinical practice related to a particular area within the scope of nursing; (2) eligibility requirements for certification through the professional society or completion of the certification process.

The purpose of the criteria for specialists in nursing practice is protection of the public. Unlike generalist nurses, who upon licensure and entry into practice are expected to be competent at least at a *minimum safe level,* specialists are expected to have *expert competence.* The public relies upon boards of nursing, through which nursing practice acts are administered under the authority of state governments, to assure its safety in regard to the general practice of all nurses. Because specialists in nursing practice hold licenses in the state in which they practice, they are subject to the legal constraints and external (outside the profession) regulations that apply under the nursing practice act.

Additionally, however, the public needs clear evidence that a nurse who claims to be a specialist does indeed have expertise of a particular kind. The profession of nursing has a social obligation to the public to satisfy that need, which it does by means of certification of specialists and by accreditation of the graduate programs that educate specialists in nursing practice. These two methods by which the public is protected against false claims are in accord with the prerogative of self-regulation (within the profession) that society has accorded as a trust to its professions. It is in the absence of such within-profession credentialing that the public turns to the law for its protection. Through credentialing of those nurses who claim competence at an expert level, the nursing profession assures the public that these claims of a higher standard of nursing competence are not false.

*If these two criteria are insufficient for certain purposes, such as for employment or reimbursement, and especially in the case of a nurse who holds a master's degree but is not certified, still other criteria can be pursued, such as are suggested in the following questions:

1. Was the graduate program *accredited?*

2. In broad outline, what was the theoretical and clinical content of the program, as described in the university *catalogue?*

3. What were the qualifications of the *faculty,* in particular those who taught and supervised the clinical work and therefore were role models? Did these faculty members hold the same or a higher degree than that toward which their students were studying, and were the faculty certified specialists in nursing practice?

50

Nursing's Social Policy Statement: Second Edition

1980

Expert competence is an abstraction—the difference between a generalist and a specialist cannot be seen until it has been made concrete through practice, over time; reliance upon credentialing of specialists by the profession is therefore a safeguard for the consumer who uses the services of a specialist in nursing practice.

Role and Functions of Specialists in Nursing Practice

Specialists in nursing practice have autonomy and freedom in practice greater than do nurses in general practice. The autonomy and freedom are based upon broader authority rooted in expert knowledge in selected areas of nursing. This expert knowledge is associated with greater self-discipline and responsibility for direct care practice and for advancement of the nursing profession. The self-discipline includes seeking periodic review of clinical data from an equally prepared expert in the same specialized area of practice.

Nursing is primarily an applied science in that it selects and applies theories from all existing sciences in order to understand and treat those conditions within the scope of nursing. In the last several decades the explosion of knowledge in all scientific fields and the development of nursing research have made monumental the task of theory selection and application in general nursing, and have correspondingly increased the risk of superficiality in this process. Under these circumstances, clinical specialization in nursing has made it possible for some nurses, through graduate-level education, to sharpen their acumen in a designated part of the whole field of nursing.

The effectiveness of the profession is increased when specialists are available to focus their efforts around a particular aspect of clinical nursing, to test application of newly available theory to conditions germane to that clinical aspect, to translate those theory applications into nursing approaches considered more useful than prevailing ones, and to assist in encouraging and speeding up the flow of new knowledge into basic nursing education and generalized nursing practice.

Characteristic functions of specialists in nursing practice include the following:

- Identification of populations or communities at risk

- Direct care of selected patients or clients in any setting, including private practice

Appendix B: Text of the 1980 Original: Nursing: A Social Policy Statement 51

1980

- Intraprofessional consultation with nurse specialists in different clinical areas and with nurses in general practice

- Interprofessional consultation and collaboration in planning total patient care for individual and groups of patients, and in planning and evaluating health programs for population groups at risk related to the specialty or the public in general

- Contribution to the advancement of the profession as a whole and to the specialty field.

It is expected of specialists that they engage in a variety of activities consistent with the aims of the specialty and the profession. These activities include the following:

- Selective participation in basic, graduate, and continuing education programs

- Participation in or the conduct of research related to the area of specialization

- Preparation of publications derived from clinical practice and related education or research that would contribute to the general advancement of practice and the profession

- Obtaining certification in the area of clinical specialization through the professional society. Such certification, including periodic review, is the profession's method of assuring the public of the validity of the specialist's credentials.

Legislation to govern specialty practice in nursing should not be sought; all nurses are governed by and liable for practice at the minimum safe levels defined in nursing practice acts. Guidelines for and regulation of practice beyond the basic level of general practice covered by current licensure should be developed within the professional association.

Specialty practice is at the growing edge of the profession, and therefore its nature and scope change as new knowledge develops. Those specialists in nursing practice who continue independent study of the problems within an area, especially through empirical research, experience many changes in role and function.

When nurse specialists are employed in health care settings, descriptions of their position and functions ought not to be standardized. The work rules for the specialist must be jointly determined and negotiated

52   *Nursing's Social Policy Statement: Second Edition*

1980

by the applicant and the employing institution. The emphasis should be on developing negotiated positions and organizational arrangements that are most likely to result in freedom and responsibility for maximum use of the abilities of the particular specialist in the particular health care setting. In joint practices and partnerships, in which nurse specialists practice on a private basis with other nurses or other professionals; joint determination of working arrangements and shared responsibility also apply.

Need for Specialists in Nursing Practice

The need of society and the nursing profession for adequate numbers and kinds of specialists in nursing practice should be monitored periodically by the professional society. While the demands of the marketplace should be allowed to regulate excess in numbers, the profession must take steps to assure that universities prepare enough specialists in nursing practice to meet needs for qualified nurse faculty, nurse researchers, and consultants, as well as specialists for direct care practice.

At the same time, the need for specialists must be balanced against the needs of the society and the profession for nurses in general practice. The responsibility of the profession and its specialists for continued strengthening of the generic foundation of nursing is a major one if fragmentation and unjustifiable costs of care are to be avoided in nursing.

Areas of Specialization

The principle applies: *Professional organizations do not initiate trends; rather, they formulate and consolidate those trends already under way within the practices of the professions in society.* Those trends that have been judged to be promising for the advancement of the profession are pertinent to determination of areas of specialization in nursing. Two major social institutions—universities and the American Nurses' Association—are involved in the establishment of areas of specialization in nursing.

Graduate programs that prepare specialists in nursing practice are initiated, established, and conducted by universities, which have the primary social responsibility for the education of scientists and professionals. Among the criteria universities use to decide that an area of specialization in nursing merits establishment of a program are the following:

1. A previously unrecognized area that lies within or would be a reasonable expansion of nursing's scope of practice is identified by one or more nurses or by another person.

Appendix B: Text of the 1980 Original: Nursing: A Social Policy Statement 53

1980

2. The nursing faculty at the university has identified through careful study that a sufficient need exists in society or in the health care system to warrant preparing nurses for that new area of specialization in nursing. Nurses who are experts in that area by reason of clinical experience, and who either have or could readily obtain the necessary credentials for academic teaching, are available. Furthermore, the expertise of nurse faculty in the area most closely related to the proposed new one could be co-opted to assist in the design and conduct of the proposed new program.

3. There is ample evidence to believe that the whole field of nursing would be diminished or limited in its long-range aim if the recognized need were ignored.

4. Funds in support of the program are available or could be obtained.

After universities have been providing graduate programs for specialty practice in nursing and accreditation of those programs is in effect, certification of specialists who graduate from those programs becomes a concern of the profession in exercising its responsibility to the public.

The American Nurses' Association has five Divisions on Nursing Practice: community health nursing, gerontological nursing, maternal and child health nursing, medical-surgical nursing, and psychiatric and mental health nursing. These divisions are interest groups; membership in them is open to any ANA member having an interest in a particular division. Each of the divisions offers certification programs for nurses in their respective fields of practice. Thirteen certification programs in nursing practice are currently offered.

Only three of these certification programs are for specialists, i.e. require a master's or higher degree in the area of specialization: the program for clinical specialists in medical-surgical nursing and the two programs for clinical specialists in psychiatric and mental health nursing. Many of the nurses who have been certified in other programs do hold master's degrees in their area of specialization, however, and would be eligible for certification as specialists if such programs existed. Many certified family nurse practitioners, for example, hold master's degrees in their area of specialization that would qualify them as specialists, although the family nurse practitioner certification program does not include a graduate degree among its eligibility requirements.

The ANA divisions on nursing practice also provide councils as

54   *Nursing's Social Policy Statement: Second Edition*

1980

opportunities for groups of nurses to meet together and share their interests and concerns related to defined areas of nursing practice.

The American Nurses' Association has recognized that most nursing practice is general nursing in a specialized area, having a specialized population or focus. Within the wide variety of health care institutions, most nursing practice occurs as a concentration in an area of nursing, based on interest, experience, and selection of employment, for example. Additionally, public interest and concern about specific areas of health problems stimulates employment opportunities that sometimes coincide with interests of enterprising nurses. Public concern also sometimes stimulates funds for short-term education of nurses, and the movement toward widespread continuing education for nurses has provided short-term concentrated education. Both of these efforts have been aimed at meeting immediate needs for nurses to work more productively in particular areas of nursing practice. Many nurses with less than graduate education have enlarged their competence for work in such areas without being specialists and without having the recognizable credentials of specialists.

As the professional society for nursing, ANA must provide structural arrangements that recognize the wide diversity of clinical expertise that exists among nurses—generalists, generalists who concentrate their practice in specialized areas, and qualified specialists in nursing practice—and thereby give recognition of and show tolerance for the difference and complexity that characterize contemporary nursing. This diversity must be seen as a constructive response of nurses to social needs in a time of rapid, complex, and sophisticated changes in present-day health care systems.

At the same time, it is incumbent upon the American Nurses' Association to provide for certification of specialists in nursing practice as a means of assuring the public that those nurses who claim to be specialists in nursing practice are so entitled by virtue of holding an earned graduate degree in the area of specialization and meeting the requirements for certification through the professional society.

Within the decades ahead, as a taxonomy of those conditions that nurses diagnose and treat is further refined, new rubrics for emerging clusters of specialization will be formulated within the profession. The American Nurses' Association must be prepared to provide structural arrangements and programming, including certification, congruent with those areas of specialization.

Appendix B: Text of the 1980 Original: Nursing: A Social Policy Statement   55

1980

Conclusion

In this statement, nursing and its scope have been defined and issues related to specialization have been presented within the social context in which nurses practice. This social policy statement is intended to assist nurses in conceptualizing their practice; to provide direction to educators, administrators, and researchers within nursing; and to inform other health professionals, legislators, funding bodies, and the public about nursing's contribution to health care.

The statement has defined nursing in terms of the phenomena to which it addresses action (diagnosis and treatment of human responses to actual and potential health problems), its use of theory to guide action, and its evaluation of the effects of action.

It has described nursing's scope of practice in terms of a boundary expanding in response to changing social needs and demands; intersections with the practice of other health professionals; a core that distinguishes nursing from other health professions by virtue of its phenomena of concern; and dimensions that characterize nursing in terms of its practitioners, its practice settings, and its accountability.

The statement has traced the growth of specialization within nursing practice, and has identified specialists in terms of criteria related to graduate education and certification through the professional society.

Nursing's social responsibility has been addressed throughout the statement—in its definition of nursing, its delineation of the scope of nursing practice, and its description of specialization in nursing. The statement is thus both an accounting of nursing's professional stewardship and an expression of its continuing commitment to those its practice serves.

56   *Nursing's Social Policy Statement: Second Edition*

1980

References

1. Page, B.B. Who Owns the Professions? *Hastings Center Report* 5:5 (October 1975), 7-8.

2. Mechanic, D. *Future Issues in Health Care: Social Policy and the Rationing of Health Services.* New York: Free Press, 1979, 6-7.

3. American Nurses' Association Division on Maternal and Child Health Nursing Practice. *A Statement on the Scope of Maternal and Child Health Nursing Practice.* Kansas City, Mo.: the Association, 1980, 5.

4. Antonovsky, A. *Health, Stress, and Coping.* San Francisco: Jossey-Bass, 1979, 123.

5. American Nurses' Association Division on Psychiatric and Mental Health Nursing Practice. *Statement on Psychiatric and Mental Health Nursing Practice.* Kansas City, Mo.: the Association, 1976, 4.

6. Phaneuf, M. *The Nursing Audit: Self-Regulation in Nursing Practice.* 2nd edition. New York: Appleton-Century-Crofts, 1976, 8.

7. Donabedian, A. Foreword, in M. Phaneuf, *The Nursing Audit: Self-Regulation in Nursing Practice.* 2nd edition. New York: Appleton-Century-Crofts, 1976.

8. American Nurses' Association. *Code for Nurses With Interpretive Statements.* Kansas City, Mo.: the Association, 1976.

9. American Nurses' Association Congress for Nursing Practice. *Standards of Nursing Practice.* Kansas City, Mo.: the Association, 1973.

10. American Nurses' Association. *Educational Preparation for Nurse Practitioners and Assistants to Nurses: A Position Paper.* New York: the Association, 1965.

11. Nightingale, Florence. *Notes on Nursing: What It Is and What It Is Not.* London: Harrison and Sons, 1859, preface and 75. (Facsimile edition, J.B. Lippincott Company, 1946.)

12. Henderson, Virginia. *Basic Principles of Nursing Care.* London: International Council of Nurses, 1961, 42.

13. New York State Nurses Association. Report of the Special Committee to Study the Nurse Practice Act, September 24, 1970, 1.

14. New York Education Law (McKinney), Article 139, Section 6902.

15. Kelly, Lucie Young. Nursing Practice Acts, *American Journal of Nursing* 7:74 (July 1974), 1315.

16. U.S. Health Resources Administration. *Instruments for Measuring Nursing Practice and Other Health Care Variables.* 2 Vols. (DHEW Publ. No. HRA 78-53) Washington, D.C.: U.S. Government Printing Office, 1979.

17. American Nurses' Association Congress for Nursing Practice. *A Plan for Implementation of the Standards of Nursing Practice.* Kansas City, Mo.: the Association, 1975, 4-5.

18. *Standards of Nursing Practice, supra.*

Appendix B: Text of the 1980 Original: Nursing: A Social Policy Statement 57

1980

19. American Nurses' Association Commission on Nursing Education. *Standards for Nursing Education.* Kansas City, Mo.: the Association, 1975.

20. American Nurses' Association Commission on Nursing Research. *Research in Nursing: Toward a Science of Health Care.* Kansas City, Mo.: the Association, 1976.

21. American Nurses' Association Commission on Nursing Services. *Standards for Nursing Services.* Kansas City, Mo.: the Association, 1973.

22. The National Joint Practice Commission. *Statement on the Definition of Joint or Collaborative Practice in Hospitals.* Chicago: the Commission, 1977.

23. Gebbie, Kristine M., and Mary Ann Lavin (eds.). *Classification of Nursing Diagnoses,* Proceedings of First National Conference. St. Louis, Mo.: C.V. Mosby, 1975, 171.

24. Gebbie, Kristine M. (ed.). *Classification of Nursing Diagnoses,* Summary of the Second National Conference. St. Louis, Mo.: Clearinghouse, National Group for Classification of Nursing Diagnosis, 1976, 200.

25. Gordon, Marjory. Implementation of Nursing Diagnoses (guest editorial), *The Nursing Clinics of North America* 14:3.

26. Bevis, Em Olivia. *Curriculum Building in Nursing: A Process.* St. Louis, Mo.: C. V. Mosby, 1978, 141.

27. Dewitt, K. Specialties in Nursing, *American Journal of Nursing* 1:1 (October 1900), 14-17.

28. NLNE Special Committee on Post-Graduate Clinical Nursing Courses. *Courses in Clinical Nursing for Graduate Nurses: Basic Assumptions and Guiding Principles, Basic Courses, Advanced Courses,* Pamphlet 2. Livingston, New York: Livingston Press, 1945.

29. Burd, Shirley F. The Clinical Specialization Trend in Psychiatric Nursing. Unpublished Ed.D. thesis, Graduate School of Education, Rutgers, The State University of New Jersey, 1966.

30. National League for Nursing Division of Baccalaureate and Higher Degree Programs. *Master's Education in Nursing: Route to Opportunities in Contemporary Nursing, 1979-80.* New York: the League, 1979.

58   *Nursing's Social Policy Statement: Second Edition*

1980

Appendix E.

The Development of Foundational Nursing Documents and Professional Nursing: A Timeline

The American Nurses Association has long been instrumental in the development of three foundational documents for professional nursing—its code of ethics, scope and standards of practice, and social policy statement. Each document contributes to further understanding the context of nursing practice at the time of publication and reflects the history of the evolution of the nursing profession in the United States. Advancing communication technologies have expanded the revision process to permit ever-increasing numbers of registered nurses to contribute to the open dialogue and review activities. This ensures that the final published versions not only codify the consensus of the profession at the time of publication, but also reflect the experiences of those working in the profession at all levels and in all settings.

1859 Florence Nightingale publishes *Notes on Nursing: What It Is and What It Is Not.*

1896 The Nurses' Associated Alumnae of the United States and Canada is founded. Later to become the American Nurses Association (ANA), its first purpose was to establish and maintain a code of ethics.

1940 A "Tentative Code" is published in *The American Journal of Nursing*, although never formally adopted.

1950 *Code for Professional Nurses*, in the form of 17 provisions that are a substantive revision of the "Tentative Code" of 1940, is unanimously accepted by the ANA House of Delegates and published.

1952 *Nursing Research* publishes its premiere issue.

1956 *Code for Professional Nurses* is amended and published.

1960 *Code for Professional Nurses* is revised and published.

1968 *Code for Professional Nurses* is substantively revised and published, condensing the 17 provisions of the 1960 Code into 10 provisions.

1973 ANA publishes *Standards of Nursing Practice*, a first for ANA.

1976 ANA publishes *Standards of Gerontological Nursing Practice*, its first such publication for a nursing specialty practice.

Code for Nurses with Interpretive Statements, is published, modifying the 1968 Code into 11 provisions and adding interpretive statements.

1980 ANA publishes *Nursing: A Social Policy Statement*.

1985 The National Institutes of Health organizes the National Center for Nursing Research.

ANA publishes *Titling for Licensure*.

Code for Nurses with Interpretive Statements retains the provisions of the 1976 edition and includes revised interpretive statements.

The ANA House of Delegates forms a task force to formally document the scope of practice for nursing.

1987 ANA publishes *The Scope of Nursing Practice*.

1990 The ANA House of Delegates forms a task force to revise the 1973 *Standards of Nursing Practice*.

1991 ANA publishes *Standards of Clinical Nursing Practice*, a revision of the 1973 standards.

1995 ANA publishes *Nursing's Social Policy Statement*, updating the 1980 work.

1995 The Congress of Nursing Practice directs the Committee on Nursing Practice Standards and Guidelines to establish a process for periodic review and revision of nursing standards.

1996 ANA publishes *Scope and Standards of Advanced Practice Registered Nursing*.

1998 ANA publishes *Standards of Clinical Nursing Practice, 2nd Edition* (also known as the Clinical Standards).

2001 *Code of Ethics for Nurses with Interpretive Statements* is accepted by the ANA House of Delegates and published.

ANA publishes *Bill of Rights for Registered Nurses*.

2002 ANA publishes *Nursing's Agenda for the Future: A Call to the Nation*.

2003 ANA publishes *Nursing's Social Policy Statement, 2nd Edition*.

2004 ANA publishes *Nursing: Scope and Standards of Practice*, which addresses advanced practice topics.

2008 *APRN Consensus Model* published by the APRN Consensus Work Group and APRN Joint Dialogue Group.

ANA publishes *Professional Role Competence Position Statement*.

ANA publishes *Specialization and Credentialing in Nursing Revisited: Understanding the Issues, Advancing the Profession*.

2010 ANA publishes *Nursing's Social Policy Statement: The Essence of the Profession*.

ANA publishes *Nursing: Scope and Standards of Practice, 2nd Edition*.

Index

Note – Entries marked by [1980], [1995], and [2003] are from the 1980, 1995, and 2003 editions, respectively, of ANA's nursing social policy statement. The page numbers of those index entries are those of this 2010 edition, not the original publications. Reproduced in this publication as Appendix B (2003), Appendix C (1995), and Appendix D (1980), their original page numbering is retained within the frame on each page.

A

AACN. *See* American Association of the Colleges of Nursing

access to health care, 4

accountability, 15, 21, 22, 30–31, [1980] 155, [2003] 99
  for actions taken or delegated, [1980] 156
  legal regulation and, 27, [1995] 128
  of patients for personal health, [1980] 140
  public trust and, [2003] 89
  See also nursing standards

accreditation of nurses, 55, 62

advanced clinical practice, [1995] 124

advanced nursing practice, 18–19 [1995] 123–125

advanced nursing roles, 19
  See also advanced practice registered nurse

advanced practice nurse (APN), 62n
  See also advanced practice registered nurse

Advanced Practice Nursing Consensus Work Group, 49

advanced practice registered nurse (APRN), 18–19, 39, 49, 50
  See also regulation of nursing practice; specialization
  certification requirements, 59–60
  certified nurse midwife (CNW), 40, 52, 54fn
  certified nurse practitioner (CNP), 39, 53, 54fn
  certified registered nurse anesthetist (CRNA), 39, 52, 54f